Copyright 2020 by Eva Penny -All rights reserved.

No part of this publication may be reproduced, distributed, or transmitted in any form or by any means, including photocopying, recording, or other electronic or mechanical methods, without the prior written permission of the publisher, except in the case of brief quotations embodied in reviews and certain other non-commercial uses permitted by copyright law.

This Book is provided with the sole purpose of providing relevant information on a specific topic for which every reasonable effort has been made to ensure that it is both accurate and reasonable. Nevertheless, by purchasing this Book you consent to the fact that the author, as well as the publisher, are in no way experts on the topics contained herein, regardless of any claims as such that may be made within. It is recommended that you always consult a professional prior to undertaking any of the advice or techniques discussed within.This is a legally binding declaration that is considered both valid and fair by both the Committee of Publishers Association and the American Bar Association and should be considered as legally binding within the United States.

CONTENTS

- Introduction 8
  - What is Dash Diet? 8
- What to Eat and Avoid on Dash Diet 8
  - Grain Products 8
  - Fruits and Berries 9
  - Meat and Poultry 9
  - Fish and Seafood 10
  - Nuts, Seeds, and Legumes 10
  - Fats and Oils 10
  - Alcohol and Caffeine 10
  - Dash Diet to Lower Blood Pressure and to Lose Weight 11
  - Top 10 Tips for Dash Diet 12
- Breakfast Recipes 13
  - Apple Oats 13
  - Buckwheat Crepes 13
  - Whole Grain Pancakes 13
  - Granola Parfait 13
  - Curry Tofu Scramble 13
  - Scallions Omelet 14
  - Breakfast Almond Smoothie 14
  - Fruits and Rice Pudding 14
  - Asparagus Omelet 14
  - Bean Frittata 14
  - Peach Pancakes 15
  - Breakfast Splits 15
  - Banana Pancakes 15
  - Aromatic Breakfast Granola 15
  - Morning Sweet Potatoes 15
  - Egg Toasts 16
  - Sweet Yogurt with Figs 16
  - Vanilla Toasts 16
  - Raspberry Yogurt 16
  - Salsa Eggs 16
  - Fruit Scones 17
  - Cheese Omelet 17
  - Berry Pancakes 17
  - Strawberry Sandwich 17
  - Ginger French Toast 17
  - Fruit Muffins 17
  - Omelet with Peppers 18
  - Quinoa Hashes 18
  - Artichoke Eggs 18
  - Quinoa Cakes 18
  - Bean Casserole 19
  - Grape Yogurt 19
  - Vegetables with Hash Browns 19
  - Berry Quinoa 19
  - Scallions Risotto 19
  - Vegetable Salad with Chickpeas 19
  - Cherry Rice 20
  - Morning Berry Salad 20
  - Sausage Casserole 20
  - Dill Omelet 20
  - Aromatic Mushroom Bowl 20
  - Cheese Hash Browns 21
  - Eggs with Greens 21
  - Walnut Pudding 21
  - Chives and Sesame Omelet 21
  - Spiralized Zucchini Salad 21
  - Millet Cream 22
  - Almond Porridge 22
  - Low-Fat feta Hash 22
  - Beans Mix 22
  - Chia Oatmeal 22
  - Pineapple Porridge 23
  - Almond Cookies 23
  - Blueberries Mix 23
  - Almond Crepes 23
  - Egg Waffles 23
  - Zucchini Waffles 23
  - Onion Omelet 24
  - Baked Fruits 24
  - Tomato Egg Whites 24
- Side Dishes 25
  - Sautéed Swiss Chard 25
  - Asian Style Asparagus 25
  - Aromatic Cauliflower Florets 25
  - Brussel Sprouts Mix 25
  - Braised Baby Carrot 26
  - Grilled Tomatoes 26
  - Parsley Celery Root 26
  - Garlic Black Eyed Peas 26
  - Corn Relish 26
  - Braised Artichokes 27
  - Spiced Eggplant Slices 27
  - Lentil Sauté 27
  - Italian Style Zucchini Coins 27
  - Light Wild Rice 27
  - Mashed Potato with Avocado 28

Baked Herbed Carrot	28
Grilled Pineapple Rings	28
Chickpea Stew	28
Quinoa Bowl	28
Sautéed Celery Stalk	28
Asparagus in Sauce	29
Thyme Potatoes	29
Spiced Baby Carrot	29
Sesame Seeds Brussel Sprouts	29
Potato Pan	29
Cauliflower Bake	30
Parsley Broccoli	30
Low-Fat Sour Cream Potato	30
Tomato Brussel Sprouts	30
Milky Mash	30
Fragrant Tomatoes	30
Baked Zucchini	31
Spiced Mushrooms	31
Garlic Broccoli Florets	31
Onion Potatoes	31
Yellow-Green Saute	31
Grinded Corn	31
Dijon Potatoes	32
Light Corn Stew	32
Shallot Brussel Sprouts	32
Basil Sweet Potatoes	32
Sweet Paprika Carrot	32
Fried Zucchini	32
Beans in Blended Spinach	33
Beans in Tahini Paste	33
Turmeric Endives	33
Sage Asparagus	33
Roasted Carrot Halves	33
Cumin Cabbage	33
Basil Corn	34
Summer Berry Soup	34
Green Beans Soup	34
Turkey Soup	34
Beef Soup	35
Asparagus Cream Soup	35
Pasta Soup	35
Black Beans Soup	35
Carrot Soup	36
Cucumber and Melon Soup	36
Wild Rice Soup	36
Green Detox Soup	36
Low Sodium Vegetable Soup	36
Lentil Soup	37
Pumpkin Cream Soup	37
Zucchini Noodles Soup	37
Grilled Tomatoes Soup	37
Chicken Oatmeal Soup	38
Celery Cream Soup	38
Cauliflower Soup	38
Buckwheat Soup	38
Parsley Soup	39
Tomato Bean Soup	39
Red Kidney Beans Soup	39
Pork Soup	39
Curry Soup	39
Yellow Onion Soup	40
Garlic Soup	40
Poultry Soup	40
Roasted Tomatoes Soup	40
Yogurt Soup	41
Fish Soup	41
Trout Soup	41
Nutmeg Soup	41
Quinoa Soup	41
Red Eggplant Soup	42
Milk Soup	42
White Mushrooms Soup	42
Cheese Soup with Cauliflower	42
Chicken-Asparagus Soup	42
Red Cabbage Soup	43
Celery and Leek Soup	43
Collard Greens Soup	43
Stalk Soup	43
Cauliflower-Potato Soup	43
Green Chicken Soup	44
Coriander Seafood Soup	44
Chicken Broth and Shrimps Soup	44
Chili Pepper Soup	44
Kale and Mushrooms Soup	44
Chicken and Sweet Potato Aromatic Soup	45
Salad Skewers	45
Nectarine Salad with Shrimps	45
Asian Style Cobb Salad	45
Tomato Salad	46
Cheese&Steak Salad	46
Corn Salad with Spinach	46

Recipe	Page
Shredded Beef Salad	46
Tangerine and Edamame Salad	46
Chicken Salad in Jars	47
Farro Salad	47
Warm Lentil Salad	47
Grilled Cod and Blue Cheese Salad	47
Tabbouleh Salad	48
Fattoush	48
Couscous Salad	48
Celeriac Salad	48
Crunchy Lettuce Salad	48
Herbed Melon Salad	49
Spring Greens Salad	49
Tuna Salad	49
Fish Salad	49
Salmon Salad	49
Arugula Salad with Shallot	49
Watercress Salad	50
Seafood Arugula Salad	50
Smoked Salad	50
Avocado Salad	50
Berry Salad with Shrimps	50
Sliced Mushrooms Salad	50
Tender Green Beans Salad	51
Spinach and Chicken Salad	51
Cilantro Salad	51
Iceberg Salad	51
Seafood Salad with Grapes	51
Fennel Bulb Salad	51
Russet Potato Salad	52
Sweet Persimmon Salad	52
Mint Seafood Salad	52
Green Dill Salad	52
Fish and Mushrooms Salad	52
Tropical Salad	53
Spring Salad	53
Tender Endives Salad	53
Bean Sprouts Salad	53
Pine Nuts Salad	53
Cucumber and Lettuce Salad	53
Endive-Kale Salad	54
Garlic Edamame Salad	54
Orange Mango Salad	54
Garden Salad	54
Dinner Salad	54
Tomato and Beef Salad	54
Avocado Sweet Salad	55
Dinner Shrimp Salad	55
Vegan Salad	55
Green Cabbage Salad	55
Grilled Tofu Salad	55
Balsamic Vinegar Salad	55
Mint Cauliflower Salad	56
Butternut Squash Salad	56
Chicken Skillet	56
Turkey Stir-Fry	56
Chicken and Low-fat Goat Cheese Bowl	57
Chicken Chop Suey	57
Chicken Packets	57
Herbed Chicken Breast	57
Chicken and Vegetables Wraps	58
Sesame Shredded Chicken	58
Chicken Piccata	58
Lean Chicken Thighs	58
Blackened Chicken	58
Grilled Chicken Fillets	59
Oregano Turkey Tenders	59
Turkey Chili	59
Turkey Bake	59
Turkey Meatloaf	60
Turkey Burgers	60
Curry Chicken Wings	60
Basil Stuffed Chicken Breast	60
Tomato Chicken Stew	61
Turkey Mix	61
Onion Chicken	61
Spiced Turkey Fillet	61
Balsamic Vinegar Chicken	61
Citrus Chicken	62
Glazed Chicken	62
Turkey Mushrooms	62
Spring Chicken Mix	62
Peach Turkey	62
Chicken with Vegetables	63
Asparagus Chicken Mix	63
Artichoke Chicken Stew	63
Creamy Turkey	63
Pumpkin Chicken	63
Chicken with Zucchini Cubes	64
Chicken Dill Soup	64
Avocado Chicken Slices	64
Chicken with Collard Greens	64

- Turkey with Bok Choy 64
- Chili Turkey Fillet 65
- Chicken Topped with Coconut 65
- Chicken with Red Onion 65
- Clove Chicken 65
- Rice with Turkey 65
- Apple Chicken 66
- Turkey and Savoy Cabbage Mix 66
- Soft Sage Turkey 66
- Thai Style Chicken Cubes 66
- Ginger Sauce Chicken 66
- Quinoa Chicken 66
- Parsnip Turkey 67
- Chopped Chicken 67
- Chicken in Bell Pepper 67
- Chickpea Chicken 67
- Carrot Chicken 67
- Turkey with Olives 68
- Chicken Tomato Mix 68
- 5-Spices Chicken Wings 68
- Onion and Curry Paste Chicken 68
- Cumin Chicken Thighs 68

Beef and Pork 70
- Herbs de Provence Pork Chops 70
- Curry Pork Chops 70
- Pork Roast with Orange Sauce 70
- Southwestern Steak 70
- Tender Pork Medallions 70
- Garlic Pork Meatballs 71
- Fajita Pork Strips 71
- Pepper Pork Tenderloins 71
- Spiced Beef 71
- Tomato Beef 71
- Hoisin Pork 72
- Sage Beef Loin 72
- Beef Chili 72
- Celery Beef Stew 72
- Beef Skillet 72
- Hot Beef Strips 73
- Ground Turkey Fiesta 73
- Sloppy Joe 73
- Turmeric Meatloaf 73
- Beef Casserole 73
- Garlic Steak 74
- Ham Casserole 74
- Beef Ranch Steak 74
- Pork Casserole 74
- Melted Beef Bites 74
- Pork Sliders Meat 75
- Beef Saute 75
- Light Shepherd Pie 75
- Meat&Mushrooms Bowl 75
- Tandoori Beef 76
- Oregano Pork Tenderloin 76
- Baked Beef Tenders 76
- Pork Stuffed Peppers 76
- White Cabbage Rolls 76
- Beef Stroganoff Strips 77
- Spinach Pork Cubes 77
- Cranberry Pork 77
- Stuffed Tomatoes 78
- Chinese Style Beef 78
- Thai Steak 78
- Stuffed Pork Loin with Nuts 78
- Marinated Beef Steak Strips 78
- Fennel Pork Chops 79
- Curries Pork 79
- Caribbean Pork Chops 79
- Bistro Beef Tenderloins 79
- Seasoned Baked Veal 80
- Balsamic Vinegar Steak 80
- Black Currant Beef Loin 80

Fish and Seafood 81
- Limes and Shrimps Skewers 81
- Crusted Salmon with Horseradish 81
- Cucumber and Seafood Bowl 81
- Fish Tacos 81
- Tuna and Pineapple Kebob 81
- Paprika Tilapia 82
- Herbed Sole 82
- Rosemary Salmon 82
- Tuna Stuffed Zucchini Boats 82
- Baked Cod 82
- Basil Halibut 83
- Tilapia Veracruz 83
- Lemon Swordfish 83
- Spiced Scallops 83
- Shrimp Putanesca 83
- Curry Snapper 84
- Grouper with Tomato Sauce 84
- Braised Seabass 84
- Five-Spices Sole 84

Clams Stew	84
Salmon in Capers	85
Horseradish Cod	85
Salmon and Corn Salad	85
Mustard Tuna Salad	85
Shallot Tuna	85
Cod Relish	85
Mint Cod	86
Dill Steamed Salmon	86
Cod in Tomatoes	86
Spinach Halibut	86
Paprika Tuna Steaks	86
Grilled Tilapia	86
Cod in Orange Juice	87
Tomato Halibut Fillets	87
Salmon with Basil and Garlic	87
Mustard Arctic Char	87
Cod in Yogurt Sauce	87
Parsley Trout	87
Halibut with Radish Slices	88
Green Onion Salmon	88
Broccoli and Cod Mash	88
Greek Style Salmon	88
Spicy Ginger Seabass	88
Yogurt Shrimps	89
Aromatic Salmon with Fennel Seeds	89
Fish Spread	89
Allspice Shrimps	89
Saffron Spiced Shrimps	89
Lemon Zest Seabass	90
Spanish Style Mussels	90
Salmon with Grated Beets	90
Cold Crab Mix	90
Onion Tilapia	90
Scallop Salad	91
Vinegar Trout	91
Fish Salsa	91
Turmeric Pate	91
Celery Crab Salad	91
Lime Calamari	92
Juicy Scallops	92
Vegan and Vegetarian Main Dish	**93**
Mushroom Florentine	93
Bean Hummus	93
Hasselback Eggplant	93
Vegetarian Kebabs	93
White Beans Stew	93
Vegetarian Lasagna	94
Carrot Cakes	94
Vegan Chili	94
Aromatic Whole Grain Spaghetti	94
Chunky Tomatoes	95
Baked Falafel	95
Mushroom Cakes	95
Glazed Eggplant Rings	95
Sweet Potato Balls	96
Chickpea Curry	96
Quinoa Bowl	96
Vegan Meatloaf	96
Loaded Potato Skins	97
Vegan Shepherd Pie	97
Cauliflower Steaks	97
Quinoa Burger	98
Mac Stuffed Sweet Potatoes	98
Tofu Tikka Masala	98
Tofu Parmigiana	98
Mushroom Stroganoff	98
Eggplant Croquettes	99
Stuffed Portobello	99
Chile Rellenos	99
Garbanzo Stir Fry	99
Taco Casserole	100
Chana Masala	100
Lentil Curry	100
Vegan Meatballs	101
Garlic Shells	101
Seitan Patties	101
Sweet&Sour Brussel Sprouts	101
Baked Tempeh	102
Marinated Tofu	102
Zucchanoush	102
Garden Stuffed Squash	102
Broccoli Balls	103
Vegetarian Sloppy Joes	103
Tofu Stroganoff	103
Turmeric Cauliflower Florets	103
Tempeh Reuben	104
Marinated Tofu Skewers	104
Spinach Casserole	104
Tofu Turkey	104
Cauliflower Tots	104
Zucchini Soufflé	105

- Honey Sweet Potato Bake 105
- Lentil Quiche 105
- Corn Patties 105
- Tofu Stir Fry 106
- Dill Zucchini Patties 106
- Zucchini Grinders 106

Desserts 107
- Savory Fruit Salad 107
- Beans Brownies 107
- Avocado Mousse 107
- Fruit Kebabs 107
- Vanilla Soufflé 107
- Strawberries in Dark Chocolate 108
- Fruit Bowl 108
- Berry Smoothie 108
- Grilled Peaches 108
- Stuffed Fruits 108
- Oatmeal Cookies 108
- Baked Apples 109
- Peach Crumble 109
- Banana Saute 109
- Rhubarb Muffins 109
- Poached Pears 109
- Lemon Pie 110
- Cardamom Pudding 110
- Banana Bread 110
- Banana Split 110
- Mint Parfait 110
- Pudding Dessert 111
- Vanilla Chocolate Brownie 111
- Walnut Pie 111
- Milk Fudge 111
- Charlotte Pie 111
- Kiwi Salad 112
- Vanilla Cream 112
- Mousse with Coconut 112
- Pecan Brownies 112
- Mango Rice 112
- Strawberry Pie 113
- Cream Cheese Pie 113
- Ginger Cream 113
- Raspberry Stew 113
- Melon Salad 113
- Rhubarb with Aromatic Mint 113
- Lime Pears 114
- Nigella Mix 114
- Peach Stew 114
- Berry Curd 114
- Cantaloupe Mix 114
- Lime Cream 114
- Chia and Pineapple Bowl 114
- Plum Stew 115
- Citrus Pudding 115
- Pomegranate Porridge 115
- Apricot Cream 115
- Cardamom Black Rice Pudding 115
- Fragrant Apple Halves 115

Appendix : Recipes Index 116

Introduction

What is Dash Diet?

The Dash diet (dietary approach to stop hypertension) is called to maintain, improve, and support the health of the whole body, and at the same time to lower your blood pressure and prevent the risk of hypertension. The diet was created thanks to the National Institutes of Health researching, and it was developed to fight with high blood pressure without medical intervention.

The main idea of a Dash diet is to decrease the amount of sodium food in your diet, but at the same time to make you eat food that is enriched with nutrients which will help to maintain the normal (stabile) blood pressure. Such nutrients are potassium, calcium, and magnesium.

The right following of the Dash diet can give you awesome results just in 2 weeks. Scientifically proved that the DASH diet nutrition plan which is correctly selected by a doctor is able to reduce your blood pressure fast in few points. The general level of blood pressure can be dropped up to 15 points per all time of the diet period.

Besides the Dash diet benefits in lowing the blood pressure, it is also a good way to lose weight and to prevent another heart disease, osteoporosis, cancer, diabetes, and stroke.

Dash diet is not the strict way of eating it is a lifestyle that can easily be followed all your life. The diet will be good for people who want to support their health and struggle from high blood pressure. If your purpose is weight loss, the Dash diet should only be adjusted by nutritionist or doctor; because in its classic way, the diet won't give the significant weight loss results.

What to Eat and Avoid on Dash Diet

Grain Products

Use only whole-grains because they are richer in fiber and nutrients. They are low-fat and can easily substitute butter, cheese, and cream.

What to eat	Eat occasionally	What to avoid
• Brown rice • Whole-grain breakfast cereals • Bulgur • Quinoa • Oatmeal • Popcorn • Rice cakes	• Whole-wheat pasta • Whole-wheat noodles	• White rice • Regular pasta • White bread

Vegetables

Vegetables are the richest source of fiber, vitamins, potassium, and magnesium. You can use vegetables not only as a side dish but also as a topping, spread, or meat-free main dish substitutes.

What to eat	What to avoid
• All fresh vegetables and greens • Low-sodium canned vegetables	• Regular canned vegetables

Fruits and Berries

The fruits and berries have the same vital benefits as vegetables. They are rich in minerals and vitamins.
The one more advantage of fruits and berries are low-fat content. They can be a good substitution for desserts and snacks. Fruit peels contain the highest amount of fiber and useful nutrients in comparison with fruit flesh.

What to eat	Eat occasionally	What to avoid
• All fruits and berries (pineapple, apple, mango, pears, strawberries, raspberries, dates, apricots, etc.)	• Grapefruit • Orange • Lemon	• Sugar added canned fruits • Coconut

Dairy

Dairy products are the main source of D vitamin and calcium. The only restriction for dash diet followers is saturated and high-fat dairy products.
Note: you can substitute dairy products with nut, almond, cashew, and soy milk.

What to eat	Eat occasionally	What to avoid
• Low-fat or fat-free cheese • Low-fat or fat-free yogurt • Low-fat or fat-free milk/percent milk • Low-fat or fat-free skim milk • Low-fat or fat-free frozen yogurt	• Low-fat cream • Low-fat buttermilk	• Full-fat cream • Full-fat milk • Full-fat cheese • Full-fat yogurt

Meat and Poultry

Meat is rich in zinc, B vitamins, protein, and iron. There is a big variety of recipes which will help you to cook meat in different ways. You can broil, grill, bake or roast it but anyways it will be delicious.
Note: avoid to eat skin and fat from poultry and meat.

What to eat	Eat occasionally	What to avoid
• Skinless chicken breast • Skinless chicken thighs • Skinless chicken wings • Skinless drumsticks • Chicken fillet	• Lean cuts of red meat (pork, beef, veal, lamb) • Eggs	• Fat cuts of meat • Pork belly • Bacon • Fat

Fish and Seafood

The main benefits you will get from the fish which is high in omega-3 fatty acids. All types of seafood and fish are allowed on the dash diet. You will find the best fish choice for the dash diet below.

What to eat	What to avoid
• Salmon • Herring • Tuna	• High sodium canned fish and seafood

Nuts, Seeds, and Legumes

This type of product is rich in fiber, phytochemicals, potassium, magnesium, and proteins. It has the ability to fight cancer and cardiovascular disease.

Nuts, seeds, and legumes are high in calories and should be eaten in moderation. Add them into your salads or main dishes, they will saturate the taste.

What to eat
• All types of seeds • All types of nuts • All types of legumes

Fats and Oils

The main function of fats is to help in absorbing vitamins; nevertheless, the high amount of fats can lead to developing heart diseases, obesity, and diabetes.

According to the dash diet, your daily meal plan shouldn't include more than 30% of fats of daily calories.

What to eat	Eat occasionally	What to avoid
• Margarine • Vegetable oils	• Low-fat mayonnaise • Light-salad dressings	• Butter • Lard • Solid shortening • Palm oil

Sweets

It is not necessary to cross out all sweets from your daily diet but it is important to follow some restrictions that dash diet provides: choose sugar-free, low-fat/fat-free sweets or replace them with fruits and berries.

What to eat	Eat occasionally	What to avoid
• Fruit/berries sorbets • Fruit ice • Graham crackers • Honey • Sugar-free fruit jelly	• Hard candy • Splenda • Aspartame (NutraSweet, Equal) • Agave syrup • Maple syrup	• Biscuits • Crackers • Cookies • Soda • Unrefined sugar • Table sugar • Sweet junk food

Alcohol and Caffeine

You should limit alcohol to 2 drinks per day for men and up to 1 or fewer drinks for women. Note: alcohol and caffeine consumption can be forbidden totally if it is required according to a medical examination.

Dash Diet to Lower Blood Pressure and to Lose Weight

Dash diet meal plan helps people to be healthier already for more than 20 years. Last few years the diet is top-rated among other popular diets. It is already proved the beneficial abilities of diet to fight with high blood pressure (hypertension). Let's give a few numbers for more conviction. According to the National Institutes of health, the effectiveness of the diet in weight loss is 3.3 points out of 5 and 4.8 points out of 5 in normalizing and lowering blood pressure.

One of the main causes of high blood pressure is the high sodium content in the human body. The salt which we usually consume is high in sodium. Excessive concentration of sodium leads to the fact that it is deposited in the walls of blood vessels. Sodium "attracts" water and the blood vessels start to swell and narrow. Consequently, the blood pressure rises and the man feels bad.

For 70 years of life, people eat approximately half a ton of salt. This is the only mineral that we eat in its pure form. It doesn't mean that salt is harmful to our body, as every mineral, it has benefits and vital for regulating the water-salt balance in the body, the formation of gastric juice, and the transfer of oxygen in blood cells. However, its excess in the diet is a time bomb for us.

Dash diet allows you to reduce the amount of sodium in your body thanks to its limitation and striking out the high sodium-containing products from your diet. The amount of sodium in day meals should be no more than 2300mg. Some research proves that decreasing the sodium amount to 1500mg can help to get rid of high blood pressure faster.

Simple restriction of sodium in the organism will not bring the desired result. The diet is balanced in the content of substances vital for normal blood pressure, such as potassium, magnesium, calcium, protein, and plant fibers. Only the right combination of these substances will give the needful effect.

The diet involves the perfect combination of different food groups such as fruits, vegetables, grains, dairy products, meat/fish/poultry/eggs, nuts and seeds, legumes, and oils. Therefore, the organism is balanced in the content of many important nutritional components.

Besides this, you start consuming less salt, sugar and fatty junk foods, which cause high blood cholesterol. If you follow the diet strictly and do sport every day, it is possible to lose 17-19 lbs for 4 months.

The biggest advantage of dash eating is that such a diet is not as fast as most radical methods, but it is natural and correct. And the lost kilos don't return back if you make such a diet as a lifestyle.

The dash diet is considered as one of the most beneficial for health. Although it is created for hypertensive patients, such a diet will improve the well-being and health of everyone.

The advantages of the dash diet are that it is recommended by doctors and is not harmful to health. The dash diet forms the habit of eating properly.

Proper diet and health care - that is what matters. And this diet is a healthy meal plan that fits this philosophy perfectly.

Top 10 Tips for Dash Diet

1. Walking is important.

Simple sports activities, walking or riding the bike will enforce the effect of the dash diet and will help in weight loss too.

The perfect combo for stabilizing the blood pressure is a minimum of 2 hours walking and 30-minute sports activities per week. If it looks complicated for you, start from 1-hour walking and 10-minutes sport exercises; increase the load till you reach the aimed time.

2. Don't change your life drastically.

To not make stress for your body, change your eating habits step-by-step until you adjust them according to the dash diet plan totally.

3. Create a food journal.

It will help you to realize how much food you eat per day and if it is dash diet-friendly. Follow such a journal should be regular. Be sure, in a week you will see a significant result in your attitude to food.

4. Make every meal green.

Make a rule to add some green vegetables to every meal. Doing this, you will provide much fiber and potassium for your organism.

5. Be a vegan once per week.

Limit your meat consumption and avoid eating meat totally once per week. Eat more beans, nuts, tofu, which are rich in proteins too.

6. Fresh box.

Make a box with fruits, vegetables, and rice cakes for your snack time. Such a box will help you to avoid the consumption of high-sodium fast food.

7. Food labels are useful.

Always read the food labels before buying packaged or processed food. Doing this, you can control the level of sodium amount better.

Notice that the low-sodium canned food should have less than 140mg of sodium per serving.

8. Add spices.

Such spices as rosemary, cayenne pepper, chili pepper, cilantro, dill, cinnamon, etc. can saturate the taste and make more delicious even non-salty meals.

9. Make your snack delicious.

People prefer different types of snacks, not all of them adore fruits and vegetables. For them, it can be a difficult step to switch on healthy food immediately. That's why make a list of your favorite products and eat them during the day like a snack. The food list will be appropriate until you get rid of all junk food from your diet.

10. Make a body examination every 2 months.

Some health problems can't be changed just by changing the food plan. The doctor's participation in your diet is important. Make the full body examination before starting a diet and then consult a doctor about any discomfort in your body or health every 2 months; it will allow following the diet in the most comfortable way for your health.

Breakfast Recipes

Apple Oats

Yield: 2 servings | **Prep time:** 5 minutes | **Cook time:** 5 minutes
- ½ cup oats
- 1 cup of water
- 1 apple, chopped
- 1 teaspoon olive oil
- ½ teaspoon vanilla extract

1. Pour olive oil in the saucepan and add oats. Cook them for 2 minutes, stir constantly.
2. After this, add water and mix up.
3. Close the lid and cook oats on low heat for 5 minutes.
4. After this, add chopped apples and vanilla extract. Stir the meal.

per serving: 159 calories, 3g protein, 29.4g carbohydrates, 3.9g fat, 4.8g fiber, 0mg cholesterol, 6mg sodium, 196mg potassium.

Buckwheat Crepes

Yield: 6 servings | **Prep time:** 8 minutes | **Cook time:** 15 minutes
- 1 cup buckwheat flour
- 1/3 cup whole grain flour
- 1 egg, beaten
- 1 cup skim milk
- 1 teaspoon olive oil
- ½ teaspoon ground cinnamon

1. In the mixing bowl, mix up all ingredients and whisk until you get a smooth batter.
2. Heat up the non-stick skillet on high heat for 3 minutes.
3. With the help of the ladle pour the small amount of batter in the skillet and flatten it in the shape of crepe.
4. Cook it for 1 minute and flip on another side. Cook it for 30 seconds more.
5. Repeat the same steps with the remaining batter.

per serving: 122 calories, 5.7g protein, 211.g carbohydrates, 2.2g fat, 2g fiber, 28mg cholesterol, 34mg sodium, 216mg potassium.

Whole Grain Pancakes

Yield: 4 servings | **Prep time:** 5 minutes | **Cook time:** 10 minutes
- ½ teaspoon baking powder
- ¼ cup skim milk
- 1 cup whole-grain wheat flour
- 2 teaspoons liquid honey
- 1 teaspoon olive oil

1. Mix up baking powder and flour in the bowl.
2. Add skim milk and olive oil. Whisk the mixture well.
3. Preheat the non-stick skillet and pour the small amount of dough inside in the shape of the pancake. Cook it for 2 minutes from each side or until the pancake is golden brown.
4. Top the cooked pancakes with liquid honey.

per serving: 129 calories, 4.6g protein, 25.7g carbohydrates, 1.7g fat, 3.7g fiber, 0mg cholesterol, 10mg sodium, 211mg potassium.

Granola Parfait

Yield: 2 servings | **Prep time:** 10 minutes | **Cook time:** 0 minutes
- ½ cup low-fat yogurt
- 4 tablespoons granola

1. Put ½ tablespoon of granola in every glass.
2. Then add 2 tablespoons of low-fat yogurt.
3. Repeat the steps till you use all ingredients.
4. Store the parfait in the fridge for up to 2 hours.

per serving: 79 calories, 8g protein, 20.6g carbohydrates, 8.1g fat, 2.8g fiber, 4mg cholesterol, 51mg sodium, 308mg potassium.

Curry Tofu Scramble

Yield: 3 servings | **Prep time:** 10 minutes | **Cook time:** 5 minutes
- 12 oz tofu, crumbled
- 1 teaspoon curry powder
- ¼ cup skim milk
- 1 teaspoon olive oil
- ¼ teaspoon chili flakes

1. Heat up olive oil in the skillet.
2. Add crumbled tofu and chili flakes.
3. In the bowl mix up curry powder and skim milk.

4. Pour the liquid over the crumbled tofu and stir well.
5. Cook the scrambled tofu for 3 minutes on the medium-high heat.
per serving: 102 calories, 10g protein, 3.3g carbohydrates, 6.4g fat, 1.2g fiber, 0mg cholesterol, 25mg sodium, 210mg potassium.

Scallions Omelet

Yield: 2 servings | **Prep time:** 10 minutes | **Cook time:** 10 minutes
- 1 oz scallions, chopped
- 2 eggs, beaten
- 1 tablespoon low-fat low-fat sour cream
- ¼ teaspoon ground black pepper
- 1 teaspoon olive oil

1. Heat up olive oil in the skillet.
2. Meanwhile, in the mixing bowl mix up all remaining ingredients.
3. Pour the egg mixture in the hot skillet, flatten well and cook for 7 minutes over the medium-low heat.
4. The omelet is cooked when it is set.

per serving: 101 calories, 6g protein, 1.8g carbohydrates, 8g fat, 0.4g fiber, 166mg cholesterol, 67mg sodium, 110mg potassium.

Breakfast Almond Smoothie

Yield: 3 servings | **Prep time:** 5 minutes | **Cook time:** 2 minutes
- ½ cup almonds, chopped
- 1 cup low-fat milk
- 1 banana, peeled, chopped

1. Put all ingredients in the blender and blend until smooth.
2. Pour the smoothie in the serving glasses.

per serving: 161 calories, 6.5g protein, 16.4g carbohydrates, 8.8g fat, 3g fiber, 4mg cholesterol, 36mg sodium, 379mg potassium.

Fruits and Rice Pudding

Yield: 3 servings | **Prep time:** 10 minutes | **Cook time:** 10 minutes
- ½ cup long-grain rice
- 1 ½ cup low-fat milk
- 1 teaspoon vanilla extract
- 2 oz apricots, chopped

1. Pour milk and add rice in the saucepan.
2. Close the lid and cook the rice on the medium-high heat for 10 minutes.
3. Then add vanilla extract and stir the rice well.
4. Transfer the pudding in the bowls and top with apricots.

per serving: 171 calories, 6.4g protein, 32.9g carbohydrates, 0.3g fat, 0.8g fiber, 2mg cholesterol, 67mg sodium, 276mg potassium.

Asparagus Omelet

Yield: 2 servings | **Prep time:** 5 minutes | **Cook time:** 10 minutes
- 3 oz asparagus, boiled, chopped
- ¼ teaspoon ground paprika
- ½ teaspoon ground cumin
- 3 eggs, beaten
- 2 tablespoons low-fat milk
- 1 teaspoon avocado oil

1. Heat up avocado oil in the skillet.
2. Meanwhile, mix up ground paprika, ground cumin. Eggs, and milk.
3. Pour the liquid in the hot skillet and cook it for 2 minutes.
4. Then add chopped asparagus and close the lid.
5. Cook the omelet for 5 minutes on low heat.

per serving: 115 calories, 9.9g protein, 3.4g carbohydrates, 7.2g fat, 1.2g fiber, 246mg cholesterol, 101mg sodium, 220mg potassium.

Bean Frittata

Yield: 4 servings | **Prep time:** 5 minutes | **Cook time:** 12 minutes
- 4 eggs, beaten
- ½ cup red kidney beans, canned
- ½ onion, diced
- 1 tablespoon margarine
- 1 teaspoon dried dill

1. Toss the margarine in the skillet. Add onion and saute it for 4 minutes or until it is soft.
2. Then add red kidney beans and dried dill. Mix the mixture up.
3. Pour the eggs over it and close the lid.
4. Cook the frittata on medium-low heat for 7 minutes or until it is set or bake it in the oven at 390F for 5 minutes.

per serving: 172 calories, 11g protein, 15.9g carbohydrates, 7.5g fat, 3.8g fiber, 164mg cholesterol, 99mg sodium, 401mg potassium.

Peach Pancakes

Yield: 6 servings | **Prep time:** 10 minutes | **Cook time:** 10 minutes
- 1 cup whole-wheat flour
- 1 egg, beaten
- 1 teaspoon vanilla extract
- 2 peaches, chopped
- 1 tablespoon margarine
- ½ teaspoon baking powder
- 1 teaspoon apple cider vinegar
- ¼ cup skim milk

1. Make the pancake batter: in the mixing bowl mix up eggs, whole-wheat flour, vanilla extract, baking powder, apple cider vinegar, and skim milk.
2. Then melt the margarine in the skillet.
3. Pour the prepared batter in the skillet with the help of the ladle and flatten in the shape of the pancake.
4. Cook the pancakes for 2 minutes from each side over the medium-low heat.
5. Top the cooked pancakes with peaches.

per serving: 129 calories, 3.9g protein, 21.5g carbohydrates, 3g fat, 1.3g fiber, 27mg cholesterol, 39mg sodium, 188mg potassium.

Breakfast Splits

Yield: 2 servings | **Prep time:** 15 minutes | **Cook time:** 0 minutes
- 2 bananas, peeled
- 4 tablespoons granola
- 2 tablespoons low-fat yogurt
- ½ teaspoon ground cinnamon
- 1 strawberry, chopped

1. In the mixing bowl, mix up yogurt with ground cinnamon, and strawberries.
2. Then make the lengthwise cuts in bananas and fill with the yogurt mass.
3. Top the fruits with granola.

per serving: 154 calories, 6.8g protein, 45.2g carbohydrates, 8g fat, 6.3g fiber, 1mg cholesterol, 20mg sodium, 635mg potassium.

Banana Pancakes

Yield: 5 servings | **Prep time:** 10 minutes | **Cook time:** 15 minutes
- 2 bananas, mashed
- ½ cup 1% milk
- 1 ½ cup whole-grain flour
- 1 teaspoon liquid honey
- 1 teaspoon vanilla extract
- 1 teaspoon baking powder
- 1 tablespoon lemon juice
- 1 tablespoon olive oil

1. Mix up mashed bananas and milk.
2. Then add flour, liquid honey, vanilla extract, baking powder, and lemon juice.
3. Whisk the mixture until you get a smooth batter.
4. After this, heat up olive oil in the skillet.
5. When the oil is hot, pour the pancake mixture in the skillet and flatten in the shape of pancakes.
6. Cook them for 1 minute and then flip on another side. Cook the pancakes for 1 minute more.

per serving: 207 calories, 6.3g protein, 39.9g carbohydrates, 3.9g fat, 5.7g fiber, 1mg cholesterol, 15mg sodium, 458mg potassium.

Aromatic Breakfast Granola

Yield: 2 servings | **Prep time:** 10 minutes | **Cook time:** 25 minutes
- 2 tablespoons avocado oil
- 1 tablespoon liquid honey
- ¼ teaspoon ground cinnamon
- ¼ cup almonds, chopped
- 1 tablespoon chia seeds
- 1 teaspoon sesame seeds
- 2 tablespoons cut oats
- Cooking spray

1. Heat up avocado oil and liquid honey until you get a homogenous mixture.
2. Then add ground cinnamon, almonds, chia seeds, sesame seeds, and cut oats.
3. Stir until homogenous.
4. Spray the baking tray with cooking spray and place the almond mixture inside.
5. Flatten it in the shape of a square.
6. Bake the granola at 345F for 20 minutes.
7. Cut it into servings.

per serving: 203 calories, 5.7g protein, 22.3g carbohydrates, 11.4g fat, 5.9g fiber, 0mg cholesterol, 2mg sodium, 211mg potassium.

Morning Sweet Potatoes

Yield: 2 servings | **Prep time:** 5 minutes | **Cook time:** 20 minutes

- 2 sweet potatoes
- 1 tablespoon chives, chopped
- 2 teaspoons margarine
- ¼ teaspoon chili flakes

1. Preheat the oven to 400F.
2. Put the sweet potatoes in the oven and cook them for 20 minutes or until the vegetables are soft.
3. Then cut the sweet potato into halves and top with margarine, chives, and chili flakes. Wait till margarine starts to melt.

per serving: 35 calories, 0.1g protein, 0.4g carbohydrates, 3.8g fat, 0.1g fiber, 0mg cholesterol, 45mg sodium, 15mg potassium.

Egg Toasts

Yield: 3 servings | **Prep time:** 5 minutes | **Cook time:** 5 minutes
- 3 eggs
- 3 whole-grain bread slices
- 1 teaspoon olive oil
- ¼ teaspoon minced garlic
- ¼ teaspoon ground black pepper

1. Heat up olive oil in the skillet.
2. Crack the eggs inside and cook them for 4 minutes.
3. Meanwhile, rub the bread slices with minced garlic.
4. Top the bread with cooked eggs and sprinkle with ground black pepper.

per serving: 157 calories, 8.6g protein, 13.5g carbohydrates, 7.4g fat, 2.1g fiber, 164mg cholesterol, 182mg sodium, 62mg potassium.

Sweet Yogurt with Figs

Yield: 1 serving | **Prep time:** 5 minutes | **Cook time:** 0 minutes
- 1/3 cup low-fat yogurt
- 1 teaspoon almond flakes
- 1 fresh fig, chopped
- 1 teaspoon liquid honey
- ¼ teaspoon sesame seeds

1. Mix up yogurt and honey and pour the mixture in the serving glass.
2. Top it with chopped fig, almond flakes, and sesame seeds.

per serving: 178 calories, 6.2g protein, 24.4g carbohydrates, 6.8g fat, 3.1g fiber, 5mg cholesterol, 44mg sodium, 283mg potassium.

Vanilla Toasts

Yield: 3 servings | **Prep time:** 10 minutes | **Cook time:** 5 minutes
- 3 whole-grain bread slices
- 1 teaspoon vanilla extract
- 1 egg, beaten
- 2 tablespoons low-fat sour cream
- 1 tablespoon margarine

1. Melt the butter in the skillet.
2. Meanwhile, in the bowl mix up vanilla extract, eggs, and low-fat sour cream.
3. Dip the bread slices in the egg mixture well.
4. Then transfer them in the melted margarine and roast for 2 minutes from each side.

per serving: 166 calories, 5.1g protein, 18.7g carbohydrates, 7.9g fat, 2g fiber, 58mg cholesterol, 229mg sodium, 39mg potassium.

Raspberry Yogurt

Yield: 2 servings | **Prep time:** 5 minutes | **Cook time:** 0 minutes
- ½ cup low-fat yogurt
- ½ cup raspberries
- 1 teaspoon almond flakes

1. Mix up yogurt and raspberries and transfer them in the serving glasses.
2. Top yogurt with almond flakes.

per serving: 77 calories, 3.9g protein, 8.6g carbohydrates, 3.4g fat, 2.6g fiber, 4mg cholesterol, 32mg sodium, 192mg potassium.

Salsa Eggs

Yield: 4 servings | **Prep time:** 10 minutes | **Cook time:** 10 minutes
- 2 tomatoes, chopped
- 1 chili pepper, chopped
- 2 cucumbers, chopped
- 1 red onion, chopped
- 2 tablespoons parsley, chopped
- 1 tablespoon olive oil
- 1 tablespoon lemon juice
- 4 eggs
- 1 cup water, for cooking eggs

1. Put eggs in the water and boil them for 7 minutes. Cool the cooked eggs in the cold water and peel.
2. After this, make salsa salad: mix up tomatoes, chili pepper, cucumbers, red onion, parsley, olive oil, and lemon juice.
3. Cut the eggs into the halves and sprinkle generously with cooked salsa salad.

per serving: 140 calories, 7.5g protein, 11.1g carbohydrates, 8.3g fat, 2.2g fiber, 164mg cholesterol, 71mg sodium, 484mg potassium.

Fruit Scones

Yield: 8 servings | **Prep time:** 10 minutes | **Cook time:** 12 minutes
- *2 cups whole-grain wheat flour*
- *½ teaspoon baking powder*
- *¼ cup cranberries, dried*
- *¼ cup chia seeds*
- *¼ cup apricots, chopped*
- *¼ cup almonds, chopped*
- *1 tablespoon liquid honey*
- *1 egg, whisked*

1. In the bowl mix up all the ingredients and knead the dough.
2. Cut the dough into 16 pieces (scones)
3. Bake them at 350 degrees F for 12 minutes in the lined with baking paper tray.
4. Cool the scones well.

per serving: 156 calories, 6.1g protein, 27.1g carbohydrates, 3.7g fat, 5.5g fiber, 20mg cholesterol, 10mg sodium, 216mg potassium.

Cheese Omelet

Yield: 4 servings | **Prep time:** 10 minutes | **Cook time:** 10 minutes
- *1 tablespoon olive oil*
- *½ teaspoon ground black pepper*
- *1 cup baby spinach, chopped*
- *3 eggs, beaten*
- *2 oz low-fat Low-fat feta cheese, crumbled*
- *1 tablespoons cilantro, chopped*

1. Heat up a pan with the oil over the medium-high heat, add spinach and saute for 3 minutes.
2. Then add all remaining ingredients and stir gently. Close the lid and cook an omelet for 7 minutes on low heat or until it is solid.

per serving: 117 calories, 6.4g protein, 1.3g carbohydrates, 9.8g fat, 0.3g fiber, 135mg cholesterol, 211mg sodium, 99mg potassium.

Berry Pancakes

Yield: 12 servings | **Prep time:** 10 minutes | **Cook time:** 8 minutes
- *2 eggs, whisked*
- *4 tablespoons almond milk*
- *1 cup low-fat yogurt*
- *3 tablespoons margarine, melted*
- *½ teaspoon vanilla extract*
- *1 cup almond flour*
- *1 cup strawberries*

1. Pour the margarine in the skillet.
2. Mix up all remaining ingredients and blend with the help of the mixer.
3. Then pour the dough in the hot skillet in the shape of the pancakes and cook for 1.5 minutes from each side.

per serving: 80 calories, 2.8g protein, 3.3g carbohydrates, 6.2g fat, 0.6g fiber, 29mg cholesterol, 60mg sodium, 91mg potassium.

Strawberry Sandwich

Yield: 4 servings | **Prep time:** 5 minutes | **Cook time:** 0 minutes
- *4 tablespoons low-fat yogurt*
- *4 strawberries, sliced*
- *4 whole-wheat bread slices*

1. Spread the bread with yogurt and then top with sliced strawberries.

per serving: 84 calories, 4.6g protein, 13.6g carbohydrates, 1.2g fat, 2.1g fiber, 1mg cholesterol, 143mg sodium, 124mg potassium.

Ginger French Toast

Yield: 2 servings | **Prep time:** 10 minutes | **Cook time:** 5 minutes
- *4 whole-wheat bread slices*
- *½ cup low-fat milk*
- *2 eggs, whisked*
- *1 teaspoon ground ginger*
- *Cooking spray*

1. Spray the skillet with cooking spray.
2. In the mixing bowl mix up milk and eggs.
3. Then add ginger and dip the bread in the liquid.
4. Roast the bread in the preheated skillet for 2 minutes from each side.

per serving: 229 calories, 15.6g protein, 29.4g carbohydrates, 8g fat, 4g fiber, 167mg cholesterol, 388mg sodium, 150mg potassium.

Fruit Muffins

Yield: 6 servings | **Prep time:** 10 minutes | **Cook time:** 35 minutes

- *1 cup apple, grated*
- *1 cup quinoa*
- *2 cups oatmeal*
- *½ cup of coconut milk*
- *1 tablespoon liquid honey*
- *1 teaspoon vanilla extract*
- *1 tablespoon olive oil*
- *1 cup of water*
- *1 teaspoon ground nutmeg*

1. Mix up water and quinoa and the mixture for 15 minutes, fluff with a fork and transfer to a bowl.
2. Add all remaining ingredients and mix up well.
3. Transfer the batter in the muffin molds and bake them at 375F for 20 minutes.

per serving: 308 calories, 8.2g protein, 46g carbohydrates, 10.8g fat, 6.2g fiber, 0mg cholesterol, 7mg sodium, 355mg potassium.

Omelet with Peppers

Yield: 4 servings | **Prep time:** 10 minutes | **Cook time:** 15 minutes

- *4 eggs, beaten*
- *1 tablespoon margarine*
- *1 cup bell peppers, chopped*
- *2 oz scallions, chopped*

1. Toss the margarine in the skillet and melt it.
2. In the mixing bowl mix up eggs and bell peppers. Add scallions.
3. Pour the egg mixture in the hot skillet and roast the omelet for 12 minutes.

per serving: 102 calories, 6.1g protein, 3.7g carbohydrates, 7.3g fat, 0.8g fiber, 164mg cholesterol, 98mg sodium, 156mg potassium.

Quinoa Hashes

Yield: 2 servings | **Prep time:** 10 minutes | **Cook time:** 25 minutes

- *3 oz quinoa*
- *6 oz water*
- *2 potatoes, grated*
- *1 egg, beaten*
- *1 tablespoon avocado oil*
- *1 teaspoon chives, chopped*

1. Cook quinoa in water for 15 minutes.
2. Heat up avocado oil in the skillet.
3. Then mix up all remaining ingredients in the bowl. Add quinoa and mix up well.
4. Add quinoa hash browns, cook for 5 minutes on each side.

per serving: 344 calories, 12.5g protein, 61.3g carbohydrates, 5.9g fat, 8.4g fiber, 82mg cholesterol, 49mg sodium, 1160mg potassium.

Artichoke Eggs

Yield: 4 servings | **Prep time:** 5 minutes | **Cook time:** 20 minutes

- *5 eggs, beaten*
- *2 oz low-fat feta, chopped*
- *1 yellow onion, chopped*
- *1 tablespoon canola oil*
- *1 tablespoon cilantro, chopped*
- *1 cup artichoke hearts, canned, chopped*

1. Grease 4 ramekins with the oil.
2. Mix up all remaining ingredients and divide the mixture between prepared ramekins.
3. Bake the meal at 380F for 20 minutes.

per serving: 177 calories, 10.6 protein, 7.4g carbohydrates, 12.2g fat, 2.5g fiber, 217mg cholesterol, 259mg sodium, 235mg potassium.

Quinoa Cakes

Yield: 4 servings | **Prep time:** 10 minutes | **Cook time:** 25 minutes

- *7 oz quinoa*
- *1 cup cauliflower, shredded*
- *1 cup of water*
- *½ cup vegan parmesan, grated*
- *1 egg, beaten*
- *1 tablespoon olive oil*
- *½ teaspoon ground black pepper*

1. Mix up the quinoa with the cauliflower, water, and ground black pepper, stir, bring to a simmer over medium heat and cook for 15 minutes/
2. Cool the mixture and add parmesan and the eggs, stir well, shape medium cakes out of this mix.
3. Heat up a pan with the oil over medium-high heat, add the quinoa cakes. Cook them for 4-5 minutes per side.

per serving: 280 calories, 14.9g protein, 36.4g carbohydrates, 7.6g fat, 4.2g fiber, 41mg cholesterol, 222mg sodium, 374mg potassium.

Bean Casserole

Yield: 8 servings | **Prep time:** 10 minutes | **Cook time:** 30 minutes

- 5 eggs, beaten
- ½ cup bell pepper, chopped
- 1 cup red kidney beans, cooked
- ½ cup white onions, chopped
- 1 cup low-fat mozzarella cheese, shredded

1. Spread the beans over the casserole mold. Add onions and bell pepper.
2. Add the eggs mixed with the cheese.
3. Bake the casserole 380 F for 30 minutes.

per serving: 142 calories, 12.8g protein, 16g carbohydrates, 3g fat, 4.3g fiber, 105mg cholesterol, 162mg sodium, 374mg potassium.

Grape Yogurt

Yield: 3 servings | **Prep time:** 10 minutes | **Cook time:** 0 minutes

- 1 ½ cup low-fat yogurt
- ½ cup grapes, chopped
- 1 oz walnuts, chopped

1. Mix up all ingredients together and transfer them in the serving glasses.

per serving: 156 calories, 9.4g protein, 12.2g carbohydrates, 7.1g fat, 0.8g fiber, 7mg cholesterol, 86mg sodium, 365mg potassium.

Vegetables with Hash Browns

Yield: 5 servings | **Prep time:** 10 minutes | **Cook time:** 20 minutes

- 1 tablespoon canola oil
- 4 eggs, beaten
- 7 oz hash browns
- 4 oz low-fat cheese, shredded
- 1 small onion, diced
- ½ teaspoon chili flakes
- 1 green bell pepper, chopped
- 1 carrot, shredded
- 1 tablespoon parsley, chopped

1. Heat up oil in the pan and add hash browns and onion. Cook the mixture for 5 minutes.
2. Add the bell peppers and the carrots, toss and cook for 5 minutes more.
3. Then add eggs, black pepper, and the cheese, stir and cook for another 10 minutes.
4. Add the parsley, stir and cook for 10 seconds more.

per serving: 290 calories, 11.8g protein, 18.9g carbohydrates, 18.9g fat, 2.2g fiber, 155mg cholesterol, 336mg sodium, 407mg potassium.

Berry Quinoa

Yield: 4 servings | **Prep time:** 10 minutes | **Cook time:** 20 minutes

- 1 cup white quinoa
- 2 cups of water
- 2 tablespoons lemon juice
- 2 tablespoon liquid honey
- 1 teaspoon dried mint
- 1 cup blackberries
- 1 cup strawberries, sliced
- 1 cup mango, chopped

1. Cook quinoa in water for 20 minutes.
2. Then add blackberries, strawberries, and mango and toss.
3. Add lemon juice, mint, and honey. Stir well.

per serving: 128 calories, 2.7g protein, 28.5g carbohydrates, 1.1g fat, 4.1g fiber, 0mg cholesterol, 7mg sodium, 201mg potassium.

Scallions Risotto

Yield: 4 servings | **Prep time:** 10 minutes | **Cook time:** 20 minutes

- 4 slices bacon, low-sodium, chopped
- 1 tablespoon olive oil
- 1 cup wild rice, cooked
- 2 tablespoons low-fat mozzarella, grated
- 2 tablespoons scallions, chopped
- ½ teaspoon white pepper

1. Heat up a pan with the oil over medium-high heat, add the bacon and cook it for 5 minutes.
2. Add all remaining ingredients and cook them for 15 minutes over medium heat.

per serving: 241 calories, 7.4g protein, 37.9g carbohydrates, 6.4g fat, 0.8g fiber, 8mg cholesterol, 91mg sodium, 65mg potassium.

Vegetable Salad with Chickpeas

Yield: 4 servings | **Prep time:** 10 minutes | **Cook time:** 0 minutes

- 1 tablespoon cilantro, chopped
- 1 tablespoon scallions, chopped

- *1 cups radishes, chopped*
- *1 apple, cored, peeled and cubed*
- *1 teaspoon coriander, ground*
- *3 tablespoons olive oil*
- *2 cups chickpeas, cooked*
- *1 chili pepper, chopped*
- *1 tablespoon lemon juice*

2. Mix up all ingredients in the salad bowl.
3. Shake the salad well before serving.

per serving: 490 calories, 19.7g protein, 69.6g carbohydrates, 16.7g fat, 19.3g fiber, 0mg cholesterol, 37mg sodium, 1015mg potassium.

Cherry Rice

Yield: 4 servings | **Prep time:** 10 minutes | **Cook time:** 25 minutes

- *1 cup low-fat milk*
- *1 cup wild rice*
- *½ teaspoon vanilla extract*
- *¼ cup cherries, pitted and halved*

1. Put the milk in a pot and add rice.
2. Simmer the mixture for 25 minutes stirring often.
3. Add all remaining ingredients and mix up well.

per serving: 201 calories, 5.4g protein, 41.4g carbohydrates, 0.9g fat, 0.6g fiber, 3mg cholesterol, 30mg sodium, 150mg potassium.

Morning Berry Salad

Yield: 6 servings | **Prep time:** 10 minutes | **Cook time:** 0 minutes

- *4 cups salad greens, chopped*
- *4 cups blackberries*
- *3 cups orange, chopped*

For the vinaigrette:
- *1 cup olive oil*
- *2 teaspoons shallot, minced*
- *½ teaspoon ground paprika*

1. Blend together all the ingredients for the vinaigrette.
2. Then mix up all remaining ingredients in the salad bowl.
3. Add the vinaigrette and shake it well.

per serving: 396 calories, 4.2g protein, 24.8g carbohydrates, 34.2g fat, 9.3g fiber, 0mg cholesterol, 28mg sodium, 326mg potassium.

Sausage Casserole

Yield: 4 servings | **Prep time:** 10 minutes | **Cook time:** 35 minutes

- *2 eggs, beaten*
- *1 onion, chopped*
- *1 chili pepper, chopped*
- *1 tablespoon olive oil*
- *1 cup ground sausages*
- *1 teaspoon chili flakes*

1. Mix up olive oil, onion, and ground sausages in the pan.
2. Add all remaining ingredients and mix up the mixture well. Roast the mixture for 5 minutes.
3. Then transfer it in the oven and bake at 370F for 25 minutes.

per serving: 73 calories, 3.1g protein, 2.9 g carbohydrates, 5.8g fat, 0.6g fiber, 82mg cholesterol, 33mg sodium, 73mg potassium.

Dill Omelet

Yield: 6 servings | **Prep time:** 10 minutes | **Cook time:** 6 minutes

- *2 tablespoons low-fat milk*
- *¼ teaspoon white pepper*
- *6 eggs, beaten*
- *2 tablespoons dill, chopped*
- *1 tablespoon avocado oil*

1. Heat up avocado oil in the skillet.
2. In a bowl, mix up all ingredients.
3. Pour the egg mixture in the hot oil and cook the omelet for 6 minutes.

per serving: 71 calories, 6g protein, 1.4g carbohydrates, 4.8g fat, 0.3g fiber, 164mg cholesterol, 66mg sodium, 109mg potassium.

Aromatic Mushroom Bowl

Yield: 4 servings | **Prep time:** 10 minutes | **Cook time:** 30 minutes

- *1 white onion, chopped*
- *1 cup quinoa*
- *1 teaspoon minced garlic*
- *2 tablespoons olive oil*
- *1 cup of water*
- *1 tablespoon cilantro, chopped*
- *½ pound white mushroom, sliced*

1. Heat up a pan with the oil over medium heat, add the onion, garlic, and mushrooms, stir and cook for 5-6 minutes.
2. Boil quinoa with water in the pan for 15 minutes.

3. Then transfer the quinoa and cooked mushroom mixture in the serving bowls. Top the meal with cilantro.
per serving: 241 calories, 8.1g protein, 31.9g carbohydrates, 9.8g fat, 4.2g fiber, 0mg cholesterol, 9mg sodium, 464mg potassium.

Cheese Hash Browns

Yield: 6 servings | **Prep time:** 10 minutes | **Cook time:** 30 minutes
- *1 teaspoon olive oil*
- *3 eggs, beaten*
- *2 cups hash browns*
- *3 oz vegan mozzarella, shredded*

1. Heat up olive oil and add hash browns.
2. Roast them for 5 minutes. Stir occasionally.
3. After this, pour eggs over hash browns and transfer the meal in the preheated to 380F oven.
4. Bake the meal for 20 minutes.

per serving: 211 calories, 4.8g protein, 21.9g carbohydrates, 12.5g fat, 1.7g fiber, 82mg cholesterol, 314mg sodium, 329mg potassium.

Eggs with Greens

Yield: 4 servings | **Prep time:** 10 minutes | **Cook time:** 20 minutes
- *½ cup low-fat milk*
- *¼ teaspoon chili powder*
- *4 eggs, beaten*
- *1 cup baby spinach, chopped*
- *1 cup tomatoes, cubed*
- *1 tablespoon margarine*

1. Heat up a pan with the oil over medium heat, add the spinach and tomatoes, stir and cook for 2 minutes.
2. Add the eggs mixed with the milk and black pepper and toss gently.
3. Transfer the pan with a meal in the preheated to 390F oven and cook for 15 minutes.

per serving: 111 calories, 7.2g protein, 4g carbohydrates, 7.7g fat, 0.8g fiber, 165mg cholesterol, 118mg sodium, 258mg potassium.

Walnut Pudding

Yield: 4 servings | **Prep time:** 10 minutes | **Cook time:** 25 minutes
- *1 cup wild rice*
- *1.5 cup low-fat milk*
- *1 tablespoon vanilla extract*
- *1 oz walnuts, chopped*
- *¼ cup of soy milk*

4. Put all ingredients in the pan and close the lid.
5. Simmer the meal for 25 minutes.

per serving: 269 calories, 8.6g protein, 43.6g carbohydrates, 5.7g fat, 1.2g fiber, 5mg cholesterol, 51g sodium, 250mg potassium.

Chives and Sesame Omelet

Yield: 4 servings | **Prep time:** 5 minutes | **Cook time:** 15 minutes
- *4 eggs, whisked*
- *1 tablespoon avocado oil*
- *1 teaspoon sesame seeds*
- *1 tablespoon chives, chopped*
- *¼ cup low-fat milk*

1. Heat up avocado oil in the pan.
2. Mix up eggs and milk and pour the liquid in the skillet.
3. Add chives and sesame seeds.
4. Cook the omelet for 7 minutes.
5. Flip the omelet and cook it for 6 minutes more over the low heat.

per serving: 79 calories, 6.2g protein, 1.5g carbohydrates, 5.3g fat, 0.3g fiber, 164mg cholesterol, 69mg sodium, 99mg potassium.

Spiralized Zucchini Salad

Yield: 2 servings | **Prep time:** 10 minutes | **Cook time:** 10 minutes
- *1 big zucchini, spiralized*
- *2 tablespoons avocado oil*
- *½ avocado, chopped*
- *2 garlic cloves, chopped*

1. Heat up a pan with 1 tablespoon of avocado oil over medium-high heat, add spiralized zucchini and cook it for 2 minutes.
2. In your food processor, mix avocado with the rest of the oil, and garlic. Blend well.
3. Put zucchini noodles in a bowl, add avocado cream and shake well.

per serving: 153 calories, 2.7g protein, 9g carbohydrates, 13.2g fat, 3.9g fiber, 0mg cholesterol, 18mg sodium, 581mg potassium.

Millet Cream

Yield: 4 servings | **Prep time:** 10 minutes | **Cook time:** 30 minutes

- 14 ounces low-fat milk
- 1 cup millet
- 1 teaspoon liquid honey
- ½ teaspoon vanilla extract

1. Put the milk in a pot, bring to a simmer over medium heat, add the millet and the vanilla extract, and cook for 30 minutes stirring often.
2. Top the cooked millet cream with honey.

per serving: 989 calories, 5.9g protein, 37.9g carbohydrates, 2.1g fat, 4.3g fiber, 0mg cholesterol, 189mg sodium, 99mg potassium.

Almond Porridge

Yield: 4 servings | **Prep time:** 7 minutes | **Cook time:** 7 minutes

- ½ cup almonds, raw, chopped
- ½ cup cashews, raw
- ½ cup walnuts, chopped
- 1 banana, chopped
- 1 tablespoon margarine
- 1 apple, chopped
- 14 ounces low-fat milk
- 2 teaspoons vanilla extract

1. Blend together almonds, cashew, walnuts, and banana.
2. Heat up a pan with the margarine over medium heat, add apple, vanilla, milk, and nut mix, stir well, bring to a simmer, cook for 5 minutes.

per serving: 392 calories, 12.7g protein, 29.4g carbohydrates, 27.1g fat, 5.2g fiber, 5mg cholesterol, 81mg sodium, 584mg potassium.

Low-Fat feta Hash

Yield: 6 servings | **Prep time:** 10 minutes | **Cook time:** 25 minutes

- 16 oz hash browns
- 1 tablespoon olive oil
- 1/3 cup soy milk
- 1 yellow onion, chopped
- 2 oz low-fat feta, crumbled
- 4 eggs, beaten

1. Heat up a pan with the oil over medium heat, add the hash browns and sauté for 5 minutes.
2. Add the rest of the ingredients except the cheese, toss and cook for 5 minutes more.
3. Sprinkle the cheese on top, transfer the pan in the oven and cook at 390F for 15 minutes.

per serving: 302 calories, 8g protein, 29.7g carbohydrates, 17g fat, 2.9g fiber, 118mg cholesterol, 413mg sodium, 523mg potassium.

Beans Mix

Yield: 4 servings | **Prep time:** 10 minutes | **Cook time:** 15 minutes

- 1 garlic clove, diced
- 1 onion, chopped
- 1 tablespoon canola oil
- 1 pound green beans, chopped
- 4 eggs, beaten
- ¼ teaspoon chili flakes

1. Heat up a pan with the oil over medium heat, add the onion and the garlic and sauté for 2 minutes.
2. Add the green beans and cook for 2 minutes more.
3. Add all remaining ingredients from the list above and cook the meal for 10 minutes more.

per serving: 141 calories, 8g protein, 11.3g carbohydrates, 8g fat, 4.5g fiber, 164mg cholesterol, 70mg sodium, 339mg potassium.

Chia Oatmeal

Yield: 1 serving | **Prep time:** 6 hours | **Cook time:** 0 minutes

- 1 tablespoon chia seeds
- ½ cup low-fat milk, hot
- 1 teaspoon margarine
- 1 teaspoon liquid honey
- ½ cup oatmeal

1. In the glass jar mix up all ingredients and close the lid.
2. Let the meal rest for 6 hours in chill place.

per serving: 33 4calories, 12g protein, 45.9g carbohydrates, 12.2g fat, 9.3g fiber, 6mg cholesterol, 103mg sodium, 398mg potassium.

Pineapple Porridge

Yield: 4 servings | **Prep time:** 10 minutes | **Cook time:** 25 minutes

- *2 cups oatmeal*
- *1 cup peanuts, chopped*
- *1 cup pineapple, chopped*
- *2 cups non-fat milk*
- *¼ teaspoon ground cinnamon*
- *2 teaspoons vanilla extract*

1. Mix up all ingredients together and transfer them into 4 ramekins. Cover the ramekins with oil and transfer in the oven.
2. Bake the meal at 400 F for 25 minutes.

per serving: 434 calories, 19g protein, 45.4g carbohydrates, 20.7g fat, 7.9g fiber, 2mg cholesterol, 75mg sodium, 644mg potassium.

Almond Cookies

Yield: 12 servings | **Prep time:** 10 minutes | **Cook time:** 15 minutes

- *¼ cup almond butter*
- *2 tablespoons honey*
- *1 teaspoon vanilla extract*
- *2 bananas, mashed*
- *1 cup flax meal, grinded*
- *¼ cup almonds, chopped*

1. In a bowl, combine all the ingredients together.
2. Scoop medium balls of this mix on a baking sheet lined with baking paper.
3. Cook the cookies at 350F for 15 minutes.

per serving: 83 calories, 2.7g protein, 10.6g carbohydrates, 4.6g fat, 3.5g fiber, 0mg cholesterol, 0mg sodium, 165mg potassium.

Blueberries Mix

Yield: 4 servings | **Prep time:** 8 hours | **Cook time:** 0 minutes

- *1 cups oats*
- *4 tablespoons chia seeds*
- *2 cups of coconut milk*
- *1 cup blueberries*

1. Mix up all ingredients together and transfer them in the serving glasses.
2. Refrigerate the meal for 8 hours.

per serving: 443 calories, 8.1g protein, 31.7g carbohydrates, 34.4g fat, 10.5g fiber, 0mg cholesterol, 22mg sodium, 475mg potassium.

Almond Crepes

Yield: 12 servings | **Prep time:** 10 minutes | **Cook time:** 10 minutes

- *1 cup almond flour*
- *1 cups low-fat milk*
- *1 teaspoon margarine*
- *1 teaspoon baking powder*
- *3 tablespoons whole-wheat flour*

1. In a bowl, mix up all the flour with, milk, and baking powder, and whisk well.
2. Heat up a pan with the margarine over medium heat, add ¼ cup of the crepes batter, spread into the pan, cook for 1-2 minutes per side.
3. Repeat the steps with the remaining batter.

per serving: 32 calories, 1.4g protein, 3.2g carbohydrates, 1.7g fat, 0.3g fiber, 1mg cholesterol, 14mg sodium, 75mg potassium.

Egg Waffles

Yield: 2 servings | **Prep time:** 10 minutes | **Cook time:** 5 minutes

- *2 eggs, beaten*
- *¼ cup low-fat cheddar, shredded*
- *2 tablespoons cilantro, chopped*
- *Cooking spray*

1. In a bowl, mix up eggs, cilantro, and cheddar.
2. Spray the waffle iron with cooking spray, add the eggs mix, cook for 4-5 minutes.

per serving: 143 calories, 12.6g protein, 1.4g carbohydrates, 10.4g fat, 0g fiber, 184mg cholesterol, 292mg sodium, 64mg potassium.

Zucchini Waffles

Yield: 6 servings | **Prep time:** 10 minutes | **Cook time:** 10 minutes

- *½ cup zucchini, grated*
- *1 cup low-fat milk*
- *2 eggs, whisked*
- *¼ teaspoon baking powder*
- *1 tablespoon olive oil*
- *2 tablespoons whole-wheat flour*

1. In a bowl, combine the zucchini with the milk and the rest of the ingredients except the oil and whisk well.
2. Brush the waffle iron with the olive oil and pour 1/3 of the batter in each mold.
3. Cook the waffles for 3-4 minutes.

per serving: 69 calories, 3.6g protein, 4.5g carbohydrates, 4.2g fat, 0.2g fiber, 57mg cholesterol, 40mg sodium, 129mg potassium.

Onion Omelet

Yield: 2 servings | **Prep time:** 10 minutes | **Cook time:** 6 minutes

- *1 oz low-fat feta, crumbled*
- *2 eggs, beaten*
- *1 onion, diced*
- *1 bell pepper, chopped*
- *1 tablespoon margarine*

1. Mix up all ingredients except margarine in the bowl.
2. Grease 2 mason jars with margarine and add egg mixture.
3. Bake the meal at 350 F for 6 minutes.

per serving: 192 calories, 8.8g protein, 10.6g carbohydrates, 13.3g fat, 2g fiber, 176mg cholesterol, 290mg sodium, 263mg potassium.6

Baked Fruits

Yield: 4 servings | **Prep time:** 10 minutes | **Cook time:** 10 minutes

- *2 teaspoons liquid honey*
- *1 teaspoon ground cinnamon*
- *4 peaches, halved*

1. Grease a baking pan with the margarine and put the peaches inside. Sprinkle them with ground cinnamon.
2. Bake peaches at 360F for 10 minutes and then sprinkle with honey.

per serving: 71 calories, 1.4g protein, 17.4g carbohydrates, 0.4g fat, 2.6g fiber, 0mg cholesterol, 0mg sodium, 289mg potassium.

Tomato Egg Whites

Yield: 4 servings | **Prep time:** 10 minutes | **Cook time:** 8 minutes

- *4 tomatoes, chopped*
- *1 teaspoon margarine*
- *1 teaspoon Italian seasonings*
- *4 egg whites*

1. Heat up margarine in the skillet.
2. Add Italian seasonings and tomatoes and saute the mixture for 5 minutes.
3. Then add egg whites and whisk it well.
4. Cook the meal for 5 minutes over the low heat.

per serving: 51 calories, 4.7g protein, 5.2g carbohydrates, 1.6g fat, 1.5g fiber, 1mg cholesterol, 51mg sodium, 346mg potassium.

Side Dishes

Sautéed Swiss Chard

Yield: 6 servings | **Prep time:** 5 minutes | **Cook time:** 10 minutes
- 15 oz swiss chard, chopped
- ½ cup of soy milk
- 1 teaspoon chili powder
- 1 tablespoon avocado oil
- 1 teaspoon whole-grain wheat flour
- ¼ onion, diced

1. Heat up the avocado oil in the saucepan and add the onion. Saute it for 3 minutes.
2. Then stir well and add soy milk and flour. Whisk the mixture until smooth.
3. Add swiss chard and stir the ingredients gently again.
4. Close the lid and saute the side dish for 5 minutes over the medium-low heat.

per serving: 33 calories, 2.1g protein, 5g carbohydrates, 0.9g fat, 1.7g fiber, 0mg cholesterol, 167mg sodium, 317mg potassium.

Asian Style Asparagus

Yield: 2 servings | **Prep time:** 5 minutes | **Cook time:** 10 minutes
- 8 oz asparagus, chopped
- 1 tablespoon balsamic vinegar
- 1 teaspoon lime zest, grated
- 1 teaspoon sesame seeds
- ¼ teaspoon ground cumin
- 2 tablespoons margarine

1. Toss 1 tablespoon of margarine in the skillet and add chopped asparagus.
2. Add lime zest and roast the vegetables for 5 minutes. Stir them from time to time.
3. After this, sprinkle the vegetables with ground cumin and add remaining margarine.
4. Bake the asparagus for 5 minutes at 400F in the oven.
5. Then sprinkle the cooked vegetables with sesame seeds and balsamic vinegar. Shake the side dish well.

per serving: 136 calories, 3g protein, 5.2g carbohydrates, 12.3g fat, 2.7g fiber, 0mg cholesterol, 136mg sodium, 254mg potassium.

Aromatic Cauliflower Florets

Yield: 6 servings | **Prep time:** 7 minutes | **Cook time:** 18 minutes
- 1-pound cauliflower florets
- 1 tablespoon curry powder
- ¼ cup of soy milk
- 1 tablespoon margarine
- ½ teaspoon dried oregano

1. Preheat the oven to 375F.
2. After this, melt the margarine in the saucepan.
3. Mix up together soy milk and curry powder and whisk the liquid until smooth.
4. Then pour it in the saucepan with the melted margarine and bring to boil.
5. Add cauliflower florets and stir well.
6. Close the lid and cook the vegetables for 5 minutes. After this, transfer the saucepan in the preheated oven and cook the meal for 10 minutes or until the florets are soft.

per serving: 45 calories, 2g protein, 5.4g carbohydrates, 2.3g fat, 2.4g fiber, 0mg cholesterol, 51mg sodium, 260mg potassium.

Brussel Sprouts Mix

Yield: 2 servings | **Prep time:** 6 minutes | **Cook time:** 15 minutes
- 1 cup Brussel sprouts, sliced
- 1 tablespoon olive oil
- 1 tomato, chopped
- ½ cup fresh parsley, chopped
- 2 oz leek, sliced
- 1 cup vegetable broth
- ½ jalapeno pepper, chopped

1. Pour olive oil in the saucepan.
2. Add leek and sliced Brussel sprouts and cook them for 5 minutes. Stir the vegetables from time to time.
3. After this, add chopped tomato, parsley, jalapeno, and vegetable broth.
4. Close the lid and cook the meal on medium-high heat for 10 minutes. Stir the vegetables during cooking to avoid burning.

per serving: 64 calories, 2.6g protein, 5.4g carbohydrates, 4.1g fat, 1.6g fiber, 0mg cholesterol, 204mg sodium, 2451mg potassium.

Braised Baby Carrot

Yield: 3 servings | **Prep time:** 5 minutes | **Cook time:** 22 minutes
- 1 cup baby carrots
- 1 teaspoon dried thyme
- 1 tablespoon olive oil
- ½ cup vegetable stock
- 1 garlic clove, sliced

1. Heat up olive oil in the saucepan for 30 seconds.
2. Then add sliced garlic and dried thyme. Bring the mixture boil and add the baby carrot.
3. Roast the vegetables for 7 minutes over the medium heat. Stir them constantly.
4. After this, add vegetable stock and close the lid.
5. Cook the baby carrots for 15 minutes or until they are tender.

per serving: 64 calories, 0.6g protein, 5.6g carbohydrates, 4.8g fat, 1.9g fiber, 0mg cholesterol, 111mg sodium, 141mg potassium.

Grilled Tomatoes

Yield: 4 servings | **Prep time:** 10 minutes | **Cook time:** 2 minutes
- 4 tomatoes
- ½ teaspoon dried basil
- 1 tablespoon olive oil
- ½ teaspoon dried oregano

1. Preheat the grill to 390F.
2. Meanwhile, slice the tomatoes roughly and sprinkle with dried basil and dried oregano.
3. After this, sprinkle the vegetables with olive oil and place in the preheated grill.
4. Grill the tomatoes for 40 seconds from each side.

per serving: 53 calories, 1.1g protein, 4.9g carbohydrates, 3.8g fat, 1.6g fiber, 0mg cholesterol, 6mg sodium, 295mg potassium.

Parsley Celery Root

Yield: 4 servings | **Prep time:** 7 minutes | **Cook time:** 20 minutes
- 2 cups celery root, chopped
- 2 oz fresh parsley, chopped
- 1 tablespoon margarine
- 1 teaspoon olive oil
- 1 teaspoon cumin seeds
- ¼ cup of water

1. Mix up margarine and olive oil in the saucepan.
2. Add cumin seeds and heat up the mixture for 1-2 minutes or until you get the light cumin smell.
3. After this, add chopped celery root and roast it for 8 minutes (for 4 minutes from each side).
4. Then add water and parsley. Close the lid.
5. Cook the vegetables for 8 minutes on medium-low heat or until it is tender.

per serving: 75 calories, 1.7g protein, 8.3g carbohydrates, 4.5g fat, 1.9g fiber, 0mg cholesterol, 121mg sodium, 324mg potassium.

Garlic Black Eyed Peas

Yield: 4 servings | **Prep time:** 10 minutes | **Cook time:** 120 minutes
- 1/3 cup black eye peace, rinsed, soaked
- 2 garlic cloves, diced
- 1 tablespoon scallions, chopped
- 1 teaspoon cayenne pepper
- 1 tablespoon avocado oil
- 2 cups water

1. In the saucepan mix up garlic, scallions, cayenne pepper, and avocado oil.
2. Roast the mixture for 1 minute.
3. Add black eye peace and water.
4. Close the lid and cook the meal on low heat for 2 hours or until the black eyepiece is soft.

per serving: 24 calories, 1.2g protein, 3.7g carbohydrates, 0.7g fat, 0.3g fiber, 0mg cholesterol, 37mg sodium, 31mg potassium.

Corn Relish

Yield: 5 servings | **Prep time:** 35 minutes | **Cook time:** 0 minutes
- 1 cup corn kernels, cooked
- ½ cup black beans, cooked
- 1 bell pepper, chopped
- ½ red onion, diced
- 2 tomatoes, chopped
- 1 tablespoon sesame oil
- 2 tablespoons lemon juice

1. Mix up all ingredients in the big bowl and leave it in the fridge for 30 minutes to marinate.

2. Shake the corn relish well before serving.
per serving: 139 calories, 6g protein, 22.8g carbohydrates, 3.6g fat, 5g fiber, 0mg cholesterol, 10mg sodium, 556mg potassium.

Braised Artichokes

Yield: 4 servings | **Prep time:** 15 minutes | **Cook time:** 35 minutes
- 4 artichokes, trimmed
- 4 garlic cloves, minced
- 4 tablespoons olive oil
- 1 lemon
- 1 cup of water
- 1 teaspoon dried cilantro
- ½ teaspoon dried basil

1. Squeeze the juice from the lemon in the saucepan.
2. Add water.
3. After this, in the shallow bowl mix up garlic, olive oil, dried cilantro, and dried basil.
4. Rub the artichokes with garlic mixture and put in the lemon water.
5. Close the lid and cook the vegetables for 35 minutes or until they are tender.
6. Sprinkle the cooked artichokes with lemon water mixture.

per serving: 205 calories, 5.7g protein, 19.4g carbohydrates, 14.3g fat, 9.2g fiber, 0mg cholesterol, 155mg sodium, 633mg potassium.

Spiced Eggplant Slices

Yield: 2 servings | **Prep time:** 10 minutes | **Cook time:** 10 minutes
- 1 chili pepper, minced
- 1 bell pepper, minced
- 1 teaspoon ground cumin
- ¼ teaspoon dried dill
- 2 tablespoons olive oil
- 1 large eggplant, sliced
- ¼ cup of water

1. In the mixing bowl, mix up minced chili pepper, ground cumin, and bell pepper.
2. After this, pour olive oil in the skillet.
3. Add the eggplants in the skillet and cook them for 2 minutes from each side.
4. Then top every eggplant slice with minced chili pepper mixture. Add water.
5. Close the lid and cook the vegetables for 5 minutes on the medium heat.

per serving: 201 calories, 3.1g protein, 18.7g carbohydrates, 14.8g fat, 9.1g fiber, 0mg cholesterol, 9mg sodium, 664mg potassium.

Lentil Sauté

Yield: 4 servings | **Prep time:** 5 minutes | **Cook time:** 40 minutes
- ½ cup lentils
- 1 cup spinach
- 4 cups of water
- 1 teaspoon cayenne pepper
- ½ teaspoon ground coriander
- 1 garlic clove
- 1 tomato, chopped

1. Put all ingredients in the saucepan and stir them gently.
2. Close the lid and cook the saute for 40 minutes on medium-high heat.

per serving: 92 calories, 6.6g protein, 15.8g carbohydrates, 0.4g fat, 7.8g fiber, 0mg cholesterol, 16mg sodium, 322mg potassium.

Italian Style Zucchini Coins

Yield: 2 servings | **Prep time:** 10 minutes | **Cook time:** 5 minutes
- 2 zucchinis, sliced
- 1 tablespoon Italian seasonings
- 2 tablespoons olive oil
- ¼ teaspoon garlic powder

1. Rub the zucchini slices with Italian seasonings and garlic powder.
2. Then heat up olive oil in the skillet.
3. Place the zucchini rings in the skillet in one layer and cook them for 1 minute from each side or until they are light brown.
4. Dry the zucchini with the help of the paper towel if needed.

per serving: 174 calories, 2.5g protein, 7.6g carbohydrates, 16.4g fat, 2.2g fiber, 5mg cholesterol, 22mg sodium, 521mg potassium.

Light Wild Rice

Yield: 6 servings | **Prep time:** 10 minutes | **Cook time:** 45 minutes
- 1 cup wild rice
- 3 cups of water
- 1 teaspoon dried dill
- 1 teaspoon dried cilantro
- 1 teaspoon ground paprika
- 1 tablespoon olive oil

1. Mix up wild rice and olive oil in the saucepan and roast the ingredients for 1 minute.
2. Add all the remaining ingredients and close the lid.
3. Cook the rice on medium heat for 45 minutes or until it will soak all liquid.
per serving: 117 calories, 4g protein, 20.3g carbohydrates, 2.7g fat, 1.8g fiber, 0mg cholesterol, 6mg sodium, 129mg potassium.

Mashed Potato with Avocado

Yield: 4 servings | **Prep time:** 15 minutes | **Cook time:** 10 minutes
- 3 potatoes, peeled, chopped
- 1 avocado, peeled, chopped
- 1 tablespoon margarine
- 1 tablespoon fresh dill, chopped
- 1 cup of water
- ¼ cup of soy milk

1. Put potatoes in the water and boil them for 10 minutes or until soft.
2. Then transfer the cooked potatoes in the bowl, add avocado and mash the mixture.
3. Add dill, margarine, and soy milk.
4. Stir the mashed potato until you get the homogenous texture of the meal.
per serving: 248 calories, 4.3g protein, 30.9g carbohydrates, 13.1g fat, 7.4g fiber, 0mg cholesterol, 57mg sodium, 940mg potassium.

Baked Herbed Carrot

Yield: 3 servings | **Prep time:** 5 minutes | **Cook time:** 20 minutes
- 2 carrots, peeled
- 1 tablespoon avocado oil
- 1 teaspoon five spices powder
- 2 tablespoons water

1. Rub the carrots with five spices powder and sprinkle with avocado oil.
2. Then transfer the vegetables in the tray and sprinkle with water.
3. Bake the carrots for 20 minutes at 375F or until they are tender.
4. Cut the cooked carrot into pieces.
per serving: 31 calories, 1g protein, 4.8g carbohydrates, 0.6g fat, 2.3g fiber, 0mg cholesterol, 28mg sodium, 145mg potassium.

Grilled Pineapple Rings

Yield: 6 servings | **Prep time:** 10 minutes | **Cook time:** 3 minutes
- 1-pound pineapple, peeled
- 1 teaspoon honey
- 1 teaspoon olive oil

1. Cut the pineapple into rings and put them in the plastic bag.
2. Add all remaining ingredients and shake the pineapple rings well.
3. After this, preheat the grill to 400F.
4. Put the pineapple rings in the grill and roast them for 1.5 minutes from each side.
per serving: 48 calories, 0.4g protein, 10.9g carbohydrates, 0.9g fat, 1.1g fiber, 0mg cholesterol, 1mg sodium, 83mg potassium.

Chickpea Stew

Yield: 5 servings | **Prep time:** 5 minutes | **Cook time:** 55 minutes
- 1 cup chickpea, soaked
- 1 onion, diced
- 1 tablespoon margarine
- 1 cup spinach, chopped
- 1 teaspoon tomato paste
- 3 cups of water

1. Put all ingredients in the saucepan and close the lid.
2. Cook the stew for 55 minutes on medium-high heat.
per serving: 177 calories, 8.2g protein, 26.8g carbohydrates, 4.7g fat, 7.6g fiber, 0mg cholesterol, 47mg sodium, 429mg potassium.

Quinoa Bowl

Yield: 5 servings | **Prep time:** 7 minutes | **Cook time:** 7 minutes
- 1 cup quinoa
- 2 cups of water
- 1 avocado, sliced
- 1 teaspoon cayenne pepper
- 1 tablespoon margarine

1. Pour water in the saucepan.
2. Add quinoa and cook it for 7 minutes.
3. Then add margarine and cayenne pepper. Stir the quinoa well.
4. Transfer it in the serving bowls and top with sliced avocado.
per serving: 229 calories, 5.6g protein, 25.5g carbohydrates, 12.2g fat, 5.2g fiber, 0mg cholesterol, 34mg sodium, 396mg potassium.

Sautéed Celery Stalk

Yield: 2 servings | **Prep time:** 8 minutes | **Cook time:** 15 minutes
- 2 cups celery stalk, chopped
- 1 tablespoon margarine
- 1/3 cup low-fat yogurt
- 1 teaspoon Italian seasonings

5. Melt the margarine in the skillet and add celery stalk. Roast it for 5 minutes.
6. Then add Italia seasonings and yogurt. Stir the vegetables and close the lid.
7. Saute the celery stalk for 10 minutes on medium heat.

per serving: 103 calories, 3.1g protein, 6.2g carbohydrates, 7.1g fat, 1.6g fiber, 4mg cholesterol, 177mg sodium, 362mg potassium.

Asparagus in Sauce

Yield: 4 servings | **Prep time:** 10 minutes | **Cook time:** 20 minutes
- 1-pound asparagus, chopped
- 2 tablespoons garlic sauce
- 1 tablespoon margarine, melted

1. Put the asparagus in the tray and sprinkle with garlic sauce and melted margarine.
2. Cook the vegetables at 400F for 20 minutes.

per serving: 51 calories, 2.6g protein, 4.9g carbohydrates, 3g fat, 2.4g fiber, 0mg cholesterol, 50mg sodium, 231mg potassium.2

Thyme Potatoes

Yield: 8 servings | **Prep time:** 10 minutes | **Cook time:** 35 minutes
- 8 potatoes, *halved*
- 2 tablespoons olive oil
- ½ teaspoon *garlic powder*
- 1 teaspoon dried thyme

1. Rub the potatoes with garlic powder and thyme.
2. Then brush the potatoes with olive oil and transfer in the baking pan,
3. Bake the potatoes at 375F for 35 minutes.

per serving: 178 calories, 3.6g protein, 33.7g carbohydrates, 3.7g fat, 5.2g fiber, 0mg cholesterol, 13mg sodium, 870mg potassium.

Spiced Baby Carrot

Yield: 4 servings | **Prep time:** 10 minutes | **Cook time:** 30 minutes
- 1 pound baby carrots, trimmed
- 1 tablespoon smoked paprika
- 1 teaspoon lemon juice
- 3 tablespoons avocado oil

1. Arrange the carrots on a lined baking sheet.
2. Sprinkle the vegetables with all remaining ingredients and bake at 390F for 30 minutes.

per serving: 59 calories, 1.1g protein, 10.9g carbohydrates, 1.7g fat, 4.4g fiber, 0mg cholesterol, 90mg sodium, 344mg potassium.

Sesame Seeds Brussel Sprouts

Yield: 6 servings | **Prep time:** 10 minutes | **Cook time:** 20 minutes
- 2-pounds Brussels sprouts, halved
- 1 tablespoon sesame oil
- 2 teaspoons apple cider vinegar
- 2 teaspoons chili sauce
- 1 tablespoon sesame seeds

1. Put the Brussel sprouts in the baking pan.
2. Sprinkle them with sesame oil, apple cider vinegar, and chili sauce.
3. Bake the vegetables at 400F for 20 minutes.
4. Sprinkle the cooked vegetables with sesame seeds.

per serving: 94 calories, 5.4g protein, 14.2g carbohydrates, 3.6g fat, 5.9g fiber, 0mg cholesterol, 80mg sodium, 598mg potassium.

Potato Pan

Yield: 8 servings | **Prep time:** 10 minutes | **Cook time:** 50 minutes
- 1 pound potatoes, roughly chopped
- 2 tablespoons olive oil
- 1 white onion, chopped
- ½ cup low-fat milk
- 1 tablespoon thyme, chopped
- ½ cup low-fat parmesan, grated

1. Heat up a pan with the oil over medium heat, add the onion and sauté it for 5 minutes.
2. Add the potatoes and roast them for 5 minutes more.
3. Add all remaining ingredients and cook over medium heat for 40 minutes more.

per serving: 99 calories, 2.9g protein, 11.3g carbohydrates, 5g fat, 1.8g fiber, 6mg cholesterol, 106mg sodium, 284mg potassium.

Cauliflower Bake

Yield: 4 servings | **Prep time:** 10 minutes | **Cook time:** 30 minutes
- 2 tablespoons chili sauce
- 3 garlic cloves, minced
- 1 cauliflower head, florets separated
- 1 teaspoon margarine
- ½ cup low-fat milk

1. Mix up all ingredients in the baking pan.
2. Cook the meal at 400 degrees F for 30 minutes.

per serving: 42 calories, 2.5g protein, 5.9g carbohydrates, 1.4g fat, 1.7g fiber, 2mg cholesterol, 235mg sodium, 266mg potassium.

Parsley Broccoli

Yield: 4 servings | **Prep time:** 10 minutes | **Cook time:** 30 minutes
- 2 tablespoons olive oil
- 1 pound broccoli florets
- 1 tablespoon lime juice
- 3 tablespoons parsley, chopped

1. Line the baking pan with baking paper.
2. Then put the broccoli inside and sprinkle the vegetables with lime juice, olive oil, and parsley.
3. Cover the broccoli with foil.
4. Bake the meal at 400F for 30 minutes.

per serving: 101 calories, 3.3g protein, 8.2g carbohydrates, 7.4g fat, 3.1g fiber, 0mg cholesterol, 40mg sodium, 380mg potassium.

Low-Fat Sour Cream Potato

Yield: 6 servings | **Prep time:** 10 minutes | **Cook time:** 20 minutes
- 3 pounds potatoes, chopped
- 1 cup of water
- 3 tablespoons low-fat sour cream

1. Boil the potatoes in water for 20 minutes and then drain.
2. Mash the potatoes and mix up with low-fat sour cream.

per serving: 169 calories, 4g protein, 35.9g carbohydrates, 1.5g fat, 5.4g fiber, 3mg cholesterol, 18mg sodium, 932mg potassium.

Tomato Brussel Sprouts

Yield: 4 servings | **Prep time:** 10 minutes | **Cook time:** 25 minutes
- 1 tablespoon olive oil
- 1 pound Brussels sprouts, trimmed and halved
- 1 tablespoon tomato sauce

1. In a baking dish, combine the sprouts with the oil and tomato sauce.
2. Bake the vegetables at 400F for 25 minutes.

per serving: 80 calories, 3.9g protein, 10.5g carbohydrates, 3.9g fat, 4.3g fiber, 0mg cholesterol, 48mg sodium, 453mg potassium.

Milky Mash

Yield: 4 servings | **Prep time:** 10 minutes | **Cook time:** 25 minutes
- 2 pounds cauliflower florets
- ¼ cup low-fat milk
- 1 teaspoon spinach, blended
- 2 cups of water

1. Mix up water and cauliflower in the pan and cook the vegetables for 25 minutes. Drain the cauliflower.
2. Mash the cauliflower, add milk and spinach.

per serving: 63 calories, 5g protein, 12.8g carbohydrates, 0.4g fat, 5.7g fiber, 1mg cholesterol, 78mg sodium, 712 potassium.

Fragrant Tomatoes

Yield: 4 servings | **Prep time:** 10 minutes | **Cook time:** 20 minutes
- 2 cups tomatoes, halved
- 1 tablespoon basil, chopped
- 3 tablespoons avocado oil
- 1 tablespoon lemon zest, grated
- ¼ cup low-fat parmesan, grated

1. Mix up tomatoes, basil, avocado oil, and lemon zest in the tray.
2. Sprinkle the parmesan on top and bake the vegetables in the oven at 375 F for 20 minutes.

per serving: 48 calories, 2.2g protein, 4.5g carbohydrates, 2.8g fat, 1.6g fiber, 6mg

cholesterol, 100mg sodium, 261mg potassium.

Baked Zucchini

Yield: 4 servings | **Prep time:** 10 minutes | **Cook time:** 20 minutes
- *2 large zucchinis, quartered lengthwise*
- *½ teaspoon thyme, dried*
- *½ teaspoon oregano, dried*
- *¼ teaspoon garlic powder*
- *2 tablespoons olive oil*
- *2 tablespoons parsley, chopped*

1. Line the baking tray with the baking paper and place the zucchini inside.
2. Sprinkle the vegetables with thyme, oregano, garlic powder, parsley, and olive oil.
3. Bake the meal at 350F for 20 minutes.

per serving: 88 calories, 2.1g protein, 5.9g carbohydrates, 7.3g fat, 2g fiber, 0mg cholesterol, 17mg sodium, 440mg potassium.

Spiced Mushrooms

Yield: 4 servings | **Prep time:** 10 minutes | **Cook time:** 30 minutes
- *2 pounds cremini mushrooms, halved*
- *2 tablespoons olive oil*
- *1 tablespoon thyme, chopped*
- *2 tablespoons cilantro, chopped*
- *¼ teaspoon ground black pepper*

1. Mix up all ingredients and transfer them in the baking tray.
2. Cook the mushrooms at 400F for 30 minutes.

per serving: 124 calories, 5.8g protein, 9.9g carbohydrates, 7.3g fat, 1.7g fiber, 0mg cholesterol, 14mg sodium, 1026mg potassium

Garlic Broccoli Florets

Yield: 4 servings | **Prep time:** 10 minutes | **Cook time:** 15 minutes
- *1 tablespoon avocado oil*
- *2 cups broccoli florets*
- *2 garlic cloves, minced*
- *½ cup low-fat sour cream*
- *½ cup low-fat mozzarella, shredded*
- *¼ teaspoon chili flakes*

1. Mix up all ingredients in the casserole mold.
2. Bake the meal at 375F for 15 minutes.

per serving: 124 calories, 10.3g protein, 6g carbohydrates, 6.6g fat, 2.4g fiber, 18mg cholesterol, 271mg sodium, 203mg potassium.

Onion Potatoes

Yield: 6 servings | **Prep time:** 10 minutes | **Cook time:** 30 minutes
- *3 pounds potatoes, halved*
- *2 onions, minced*
- *2 tablespoons olive oil*
- *1 teaspoon thyme, dried*
- *1/3 cup low-fat parmesan, grated*
- *2 tablespoons margarine, melted*

1. Rub the potato halves with minced onion and thyme.
2. Then sprinkle them with olive oil and thyme and transfer in the baking tray.
3. Cook the potatoes at 400 F for 30 minutes.
4. Sprinkle the cooked vegetables with margarine.

per serving: 260 calories, 5.4g protein, 39.3g carbohydrates, 9.8g fat, 6.3g fiber, 5mg cholesterol, 145mg sodium, 987mg potassium.

Yellow-Green Saute

Yield: 2 servings | **Prep time:** 8 minutes | **Cook time:** 15 minutes
- *1 cup corn kernels, cooked*
- *2 cups spinach, chopped*
- *1 teaspoon smoked paprika*
- *½ cup fresh cilantro, chopped*
- *1 tablespoon margarine*
- *¼ cup of water*

1. Heat up a pan with the margarine over medium-high heat, add the corn, spinach, and all remaining ingredients, toss, cook over medium heat for 10 minutes.
2. Stir the meal well.

per serving: 128 calories, 3.7g protein, 16.4g carbohydrates, 6.9g fat, 3.3g fiber, 0mg cholesterol, 105mg sodium, 424mg potassium.

Grinded Corn

Yield: 4 servings | **Prep time:** 10 minutes | **Cook time:** 15 minutes
- *2 cups corn kernels, grinded*
- *1 yellow onion, chopped*

- ½ cup of soy milk
- 1 teaspoon cayenne pepper
- 1 teaspoon margarine

1. Heat up a pan over medium-high heat, add margarine and melt it.
2. Add corn, onion, cayenne pepper and stir and cook for 8 minutes.
3. Add soy milk and cork kernels. Simmer the meal for 5 minutes on low heat.

per serving: 103 calories, 3.9g protein, 19.3g carbohydrates, 2.5g fat, 3g fiber, 0mg cholesterol, 39mg sodium, 294mg potassium.

Dijon Potatoes

Yield: 4 servings | **Prep time:** 5 minutes | **Cook time:** 60 minutes

- 2 cups potatoes, peeled and cut into wedges
- 2 tablespoons olive oil
- 1 tablespoon Dijon mustard
- 1 teaspoon minced garlic

1. In a baking pan, combine the potatoes with all remaining ingredients and transfer in the preheated to 400F oven.
2. Bake the meal for 60 minutes.

per serving: 115 calories, 1.5g protein, 12.2g carbohydrates, 7.2g fat, 1.9g fiber, 0mg cholesterol, 49mg sodium, 313mg potassium.

Light Corn Stew

Yield: 4 servings | **Prep time:** 10 minutes | **Cook time:** 12 minutes

- 4 cups corn kernels
- 1 cup collard greens, chopped
- ½ teaspoon smoked paprika
- ¼ cup low-fat milk
- 3 oz scallions, chopped

1. Put al ingredients in the saucepan, stir well, and close the lid.
2. Cook the stew for 12 minutes on the medium heat.

per serving: 149 calories, 6.2g protein, 32.1g carbohydrates, 2.1g fat, 5.2g fiber, 1mg cholesterol, 35mg sodium, 504mg potassium.

Shallot Brussel Sprouts

Yield: 4 servings | **Prep time:** 5 minutes | **Cook time:** 30 minutes

- 1 pound Brussels sprouts, trimmed and halved
- 1 tablespoon canola oil
- 2 shallots, chopped
- ¼ teaspoon ground black pepper
- ¼ cup low-fat sour cream
- ½ cup cashews, chopped

1. Heat up olive oil in the pan and add all ingredients from the list above. Mix up them well.
2. Then transfer the pan in the oven and cook the meal at 355F for 30 minutes.

per serving: 196 calories, 7g protein, 17.6g carbohydrates, 12.8g fat, 4.8g fiber, 3mg cholesterol, 44mg sodium, 541mg potassium.

Basil Sweet Potatoes

Yield: 4 servings | **Prep time:** 10 minutes | **Cook time:** 60 minutes

- 4 sweet potatoes, sliced
- 1 tablespoon olive oil
- 1 teaspoon ground black pepper
- 1 teaspoon dried basil
- 2 tablespoons low-fat yogurt
- ½ teaspoon cilantro, chopped

1. Put the sweet potatoes in the baking tray and sprinkle with olive oil, ground black pepper, basil, and cilantro.
2. Bake them in the preheated to 400F oven for 60 minutes.
3. Sprinkle the cooked sweet potatoes with low-fat yogurt.

per serving: 217 calories, 0.5g protein, 2g 2.9carbohydrates, 13.6g fat, 4.1g fiber, 0mg cholesterol, 226mg sodium, 25mg potassium.

Sweet Paprika Carrot

Yield: 4 servings | **Prep time:** 10 minutes | **Cook time:** 30 minutes

- 2 tablespoons olive oil
- 1 pound carrots, peeled and roughly cubed
- 1 white onion, chopped
- 1 tablespoon sweet paprika

1. Put the carrot in the baking tray, add all remaining ingredients and shale well.
2. Bake the carrots at 380F for 30 minutes.

per serving: 122 calories, 1.5g protein, 14.7g carbohydrates, 7.3g fat, 4g fiber, 0mg cholesterol, 80mg sodium, 443mg potassium.

Fried Zucchini

Yield: 4 servings | **Prep time:** 10 minutes | **Cook time:** 20 minutes
- 4 zucchinis, cut into fries
- ½ teaspoon ground black pepper
- 1 tablespoon olive oil
- ¼ teaspoon onion powder

1. Line the baking tray with baking paper and arrange the zucchini inside.
2. Sprinkle them with ground black pepper, olive oil, and onion powder.
3. Bake the vegetables at 400F for 20 minutes.

per serving: 63 calories, 2.4g protein, 6.9g carbohydrates, 3.9g fat, 2.2g fiber, 0mg cholesterol, 20mg sodium, 518mg potassium.

Beans in Blended Spinach

Yield: 4 servings | **Prep time:** 10 minutes | **Cook time:** 15 minutes
- ½ cup fresh spinach, blended
- 2 teaspoons smoked paprika
- 2 cups green beans, chopped
- 1 tablespoon lime juice
- 2 tablespoons avocado oil

1. Heat up a pan with the oil over medium-high heat.
2. Add the beans and all the remaining ingredients.
3. Cook them for 15 minutes over the medium heat.

per serving: 31 calories, 1.4g protein, 5.3g carbohydrates, 1.1g fat, 2.7g fiber, 0mg cholesterol, 8mg sodium, 186mg potassium.

Beans in Tahini Paste

Yield: 2 servings | **Prep time:** 8 minutes | **Cook time:** 15 minutes
- 2 tablespoons tahini paste
- 1 tablespoon lemon juice
- 2 tablespoons olive oil
- 1 garlic clove, minced
- 10 ounces green beans, halved
- ½ teaspoon white pepper

1. Mix up lemon juice, tahini, and white pepper. Whisk well.
2. Heat up a pan with the oil over medium-high heat, add garlic, stir and cook for 1 minute.
3. Add the green beans, toss and cook for 14 minutes.
4. Add tahini dressing, toss and transfer in the serving plates.

per serving: 259 calories, 5.4g protein, 14.3g carbohydrates, 22.3g fat, 6.4g fiber, 0mg cholesterol, 28mg sodium, 381mg potassium.

Turmeric Endives

Yield: 4 servings | **Prep time:** 10 minutes | **Cook time:** 20 minutes
- 2 endives, halved lengthwise
- 2 tablespoons olive oil
- ½ teaspoon turmeric powder

1. In a baking pan, combine the endives and all remaining ingredients.
2. Bake the meal at 400 F for 20 minutes.

per serving: 105 calories, 3.2g protein, 8.8g carbohydrates, 7.5g fat, 8g fiber, 0mg cholesterol, 57mg sodium, 812mg potassium.

Sage Asparagus

Yield: 4 servings | **Prep time:** 10 minutes | **Cook time:** 6 minutes
- 2 pounds asparagus, trimmed
- 2 tablespoons canola oil
- 1 teaspoon dried sage

1. Mix up asparagus, oil, and sage.
2. Transfer the vegetables in the grill and cook for 3 minutes at 400 F.

per serving: 108 calories, 5g protein, 8.9g carbohydrates, 7.3g fat, 4.8g fiber, 0mg cholesterol, 5mg sodium, 460mg potassium.

Roasted Carrot Halves

Yield: 4 servings | **Prep time:** 10 minutes | **Cook time:** 30 minutes
- 2 pounds carrots, halved
- ½ teaspoon dried cilantro
- 3 tablespoons olive oil

1. Put the carrots in the baking pan, sprinkle with olive oil and dried cilantro.
2. Bake the carrots at 390F for 25 minutes.

per serving: 183 calories, 1.9g protein, 22.3g carbohydrates, 10.5g fat, 5.6g fiber, 0mg cholesterol, 156mg sodium, 725mg potassium.

Cumin Cabbage

Yield: 4 servings | **Prep time:** 10 minutes | **Cook time:** 20 minutes

- 1 pound white cabbage, roughly shredded
- 2 tablespoons olive oil
- 1 onion, chopped
- 2 garlic cloves, minced
- 2 tablespoons balsamic vinegar
- 1 teaspoon cumin seeds

1. Heat up a pan with the oil over medium heat, add the onion and sauté for 5 minutes.
2. Add the cabbage and all the remaining ingredients.
3. Stir well and cook the meal over medium heat for 15 minutes.

per serving: 105 calories, 1.9g protein, 10g carbohydrates, 7.3g fat, 3.5g fiber, 0mg cholesterol, 23mg sodium, 254mg potassium.

Basil Corn

Yield: 4 servings | **Prep time:** 10 minutes | **Cook time:** 15 minutes

- 1 cup corn kernels
- 2 oz basil, chopped
- 1 tablespoon olive oil
- 1 yellow onion, chopped
- ½ teaspoon red pepper flakes

1. Heat up a pan with the oil over medium-high heat, add the onion, stir and sauté for 5 minutes.
2. Then add all remaining ingredients, stir well and cook for 10 minutes more over the medium heat.

per serving: 78 calories, 2g protein, 10.3g carbohydrates, 4.1g fat, 1.9g fiber, 0mg cholesterol, 7mg sodium, 191mg potassium.

Soups

Summer Berry Soup

Yield: 2 servings | **Prep time:** 10 minutes | **Cook time:** 10 minutes

- ½ cup apple juice
- ¼ cup strawberries
- ¼ cup raspberries
- ¼ cup blackberries
- ¼ cup blueberries
- 1 teaspoon potato starch
- ¼ teaspoon ground cinnamon

1. Pour apple juice in the saucepan.
2. Add all berries and ground cinnamon. Close the lid and bring ingredients to boil.
3. Pour 3 tablespoons of apple juice mixture in the glass, add potato starch and whisk it until smooth.
4. Then pour the starch mixture in the berry soup and stir until the soup is thickened.
5. Close the lid and leave the soup to rest for 10 minutes.

per serving: 71 calories, 0.8g protein, 17.3g carbohydrates, 0.4g fat, 3g fiber, 0mg cholesterol, 3mg sodium, 158mg potassium.

Green Beans Soup

Yield: 4 servings | **Prep time:** 5 minutes | **Cook time:** 40 minutes

- ½ onion, diced
- 1/3 cup green beans, soaked
- 3 cups of water
- ½ sweet pepper, chopped
- 2 potatoes, chopped
- 1 tablespoon fresh cilantro, chopped
- 1 teaspoon chili flakes

1. Put all ingredients in the saucepan and close the lid.
2. Cook the soup on medium heat for 40 minutes or until all ingredients are soft.

per serving: 87 calories, 2.3g protein, 19.8g carbohydrates, 0.2g fat, 3.4g fiber, 0mg cholesterol, 13mg sodium, 505mg potassium.

Turkey Soup

Yield: 3 servings | **Prep time:** 10 minutes | **Cook time:** 25 minutes

- 1 potato, diced
- 1 cup ground turkey
- 1 teaspoon cayenne pepper
- 1 onion, diced
- 1 tablespoon olive oil
- ¼ carrot, diced
- 2 cups of water

1. Heat up olive oil in the saucepan and add diced onion and carrot.
2. Cook the vegetables for 3 minutes. Then stir them well and add ground turkey and cayenne pepper.
3. Add diced potato and stir the ingredients well. Cook them for 2 minutes more.
4. Then add water. Check if you put all the ingredients.
5. Close the lid and cook soup for 20 minutes.

per serving: 317 calories, 31.8g protein, 14.2g carbohydrates, 16.9g fat, 2.3g fiber, 112mg cholesterol, 131mg sodium, 619mg potassium.

Beef Soup

Yield: 4 servings | **Prep time:** 7 minutes | **Cook time:** 45 minutes
- 1-pound beef sirloin, chopped
- 4 oz leek, chopped
- 1 tablespoon margarine
- 1 teaspoon chili powder
- 1 potato, chopped
- 3 cups of water

1. Toss margarine in the saucepan and melt it.
2. Add chopped beef sirloin, chili powder, and leek. Cook the ingredients for 4 minutes (for 2 minutes per side).
3. After this, add chopped potato and water. Close the lid.
4. Cook the beef soup for 40 minutes on medium heat.

per serving: 288 calories, 35.8g protein, 11.8g carbohydrates, 10.2g fat, 1.7g fiber, 101mg cholesterol, 128mg sodium, 702mg potassium.

Asparagus Cream Soup

Yield: 2 servings | **Prep time:** 5 minutes | **Cook time:** 30 minutes
- 2 cups low-sodium chicken stock
- 1 cup asparagus, chopped
- 2 tablespoons low-fat sour cream
- 1 teaspoon dried oregano
- 1 garlic clove, diced
- 1 teaspoon olive oil
- 1 cup broccoli, chopped

1. Pour olive oil in the saucepan and heat it up for 1 minute. Add garlic and roast it for 1 minute more.
2. After this, add all remaining ingredients from the list above and close the lid.
3. Simmer the soup for 25 minutes.
4. Then blend the soup with the help of the immersion blender until smooth.
5. Simmer the soup for 3 minutes more.

per serving: 38 calories, 2.2g protein, 4.1g carbohydrates, 1.8g fat, 1.5g fiber, 1mg cholesterol, 82mg sodium, 149mg potassium.

Pasta Soup

Yield: 2 servings | **Prep time:** 5 minutes | **Cook time:** 13 minutes
- 2 oz whole-grain pasta
- ½ cup corn kernels
- 1 oz carrot, shredded
- 3 oz celery stalk, chopped
- 2 cups low-sodium chicken stock
- 1 teaspoon ground black pepper

1. Bring the chicken stock to boil and add shredded carrot and celery stalk. Simmer the liquid for 5 minutes.
2. After this, add corn kernels, ground black pepper, and pasta. Stir the soup well.
3. Simmer it on the medium heat for 8 minutes.

per serving: 263 calories, 11.8g protein, 49.6g carbohydrates, 2.6g fat, 9.4g fiber, 0mg cholesterol, 200mg sodium, 273mg potassium.

Black Beans Soup

Yield: 6 servings | **Prep time:** 8 minutes | **Cook time:** 25 minutes
- 2 cups black beans, cooked
- 1 yellow onion, diced
- ¼ cup sweet pepper, chopped
- 5 cups low-sodium chicken broth
- 1 carrot, shredded
- 1 teaspoon dried oregano
- ½ teaspoon ground cumin
- 1 teaspoon chili flakes
- ½ cup fresh cilantro, chopped
- 1 tablespoon avocado oil

1. Pour avocado oil in the saucepan and add shredded carrot and onion. Cook the vegetables for 4 minutes. Stir them from time to time.
2. After this, add sweet pepper, black beans, oregano, and all the remaining ingredients.
3. Close the lid and cook the soup on medium heat for 15 minutes.
4. After this, blend the soup for 1 minute with the help of the immersion blender. The cooked soup should be totally smooth.
5. Simmer it for 1 minute more.

per serving: 251 calories, 16.1g protein, 44.7g carbohydrates, 1.3g fat, 10.8g fiber,

0mg cholesterol, 71mg sodium, 1050mg potassium.

Carrot Soup

Yield: 3 servings | **Prep time:** 10 minutes | **Cook time:** 35 minutes
- 1 cup carrot, shredded
- 1 teaspoon curry paste
- 1 tablespoon olive oil
- 1 yellow onion, diced
- ½ teaspoon chili flakes
- 1 tablespoon lemon juice
- 2 cups low-sodium chicken broth

1. Heat up olive oil in the saucepan and add the onion. Cook it until light brown.
2. Add grated carrot, curry paste, chili flakes, and chicken broth.
3. Close the lid and cook the soup for 25 minutes.
4. Then blend it with the help of the immersion blender until smooth.
5. Add lemon juice and cook the soup for 5 minutes more.

per serving: 92 calories, 2.2g protein, 8.3g carbohydrates, 5.7g fat, 1.7g fiber, 0mg cholesterol, 74mg sodium, 178mg potassium.

Cucumber and Melon Soup

Yield: 4 servings | **Prep time:** 25 minutes | **Cook time:** 0 minutes
- 4 cucumbers, chopped
- 9 oz melon, chopped
- ½ cup fresh cilantro, chopped
- 1 teaspoon honey
- 2 tablespoons lemon juice
- ½ teaspoon cayenne pepper

1. Put all ingredients in the blender and blend until smooth.
2. Transfer the smooth soup in the serving bowls and refrigerate for 15 minutes before serving.

per serving: 75 calories, 2.6g protein, 17.9g carbohydrates, 0.6g fat, 2.2g fiber, 0mg cholesterol, 19mg sodium, 638mg potassium.

Wild Rice Soup

Yield: 2 servings | **Prep time:** 10 minutes | **Cook time:** 30 minutes
- ¼ cup wild rice
- 2 cups low-sodium chicken broth
- 1 potato, chopped
- 1 teaspoon ground turmeric
- ¼ teaspoon dried dill
- 1 tablespoon low-fat sour cream

1. Pour chicken broth in the saucepan and bring it to boil.
2. Add wild rice and cook it for 10 minutes.
3. After this, add potato, turmeric, dill, and low-fat sour cream.
4. Close the lid and cook the soup for 20 minutes.

per serving: 171 calories, 7.3g protein, 32.6g carbohydrates, 1.4g fat, 3.4g fiber, 3mg cholesterol, 100mg sodium, 475mg potassium.

Green Detox Soup

Yield: 4 servings | **Prep time:** 10 minutes | **Cook time:** 12 minutes
- 1 onion, diced
- 1 large zucchini, chopped
- 1 teaspoon fresh mint, chopped
- ½ cup celery stalk, chopped
- 1 teaspoon ground paprika
- 1 tablespoon olive oil
- 2 tablespoons lime juice
- 1 cup low-fat yogurt

1. Heat up olive oil in the saucepan.
2. Add diced onion and cook it for 2 minutes. Stir it well.
3. Add zucchini, mint, and celery stalk.
4. Cook the vegetables for 10 minutes. Stir them from time to time.
5. After this, add lime juice and ground paprika.
6. Blend the vegetables with the help of the immersion blender and remove them from the heat.
7. Add yogurt and stir the soup well.

per serving: 103 calories, 5protein, 10.8g carbohydrates, 4.5g fat, 1.9g fiber, 4mg cholesterol, 64mg sodium, 448mg potassium.

Low Sodium Vegetable Soup

Yield: 3 servings | **Prep time:** 10 minutes | **Cook time:** 15 minutes
- 3 cups low-sodium vegetable broth
- ½ cup spinach, chopped
- 1/3 cup broccoli, chopped
- 2 potatoes, chopped
- ¼ cup low-fat yogurt
- 2 oz green beans, cooked
- 1 teaspoon cayenne pepper

- 1 tomato, roughly chopped
1. Pour vegetable broth in the saucepan and bring it to boil.
2. Add potatoes, cayenne pepper, and green beans.
3. Bring the ingredients to boil and simmer for 5 minutes.
4. After this, add spinach, yogurt, broccoli, and tomato.
5. Simmer the soup for 10 minutes.

per serving: 144 calories, 6.6g protein, 28.1g carbohydrates, 0.6g fat, 4.8g fiber, 1mg cholesterol, 102mg sodium, 786mg potassium.

Lentil Soup

Yield: 4 servings | **Prep time:** 10 minutes | **Cook time:** 20 minutes
- ½ onion, diced
- 1 cup lentils
- 7 cups low-sodium chicken broth
- 1 teaspoon chili flakes
- ½ teaspoon chili powder
- 1 bell pepper, chopped
- 1 tablespoon margarine
- 1 tablespoon tomato paste

1. Toss margarine in the saucepan and melt it.
2. Then add bell pepper and onion. Cook the vegetables until the onion is light brown.
3. After this, add lentil and tomato paste. Mix up the ingredients.
4. Add chicken broth, chili powder, and chili flakes.
5. Stir the soup well and close the lid.
6. Cook the soup for 15 minutes on medium heat.

per serving: 240 calories, 16.6g protein, 35.1g carbohydrates, 3.5g fat, 15.6g fiber, 0mg cholesterol, 167mg sodium, 584mg potassium.

Pumpkin Cream Soup

Yield: 5 servings | **Prep time:** 10 minutes | **Cook time:** 20 minutes
- 1-pound pumpkin, chopped
- 1 teaspoon ground cumin
- ½ cup cauliflower, chopped
- 4 cups of water
- 1 teaspoon ground turmeric
- ½ teaspoon ground nutmeg
- 1 tablespoon fresh dill, chopped
- 1 teaspoon olive oil
- ½ cup skim milk

1. Roast the pumpkin with olive oil in the saucepan for 3 minutes.
2. Then stir well and add cauliflower, cumin, turmeric, nutmeg, and water.
3. Close the lid and cook the soup on medium mode for 15 minutes or until the pumpkin is soft.
4. Then blend the mixture until smooth and add skim milk. Remove the soup from heat and top with dill.

per serving: 56 calories, 2.2g protein, 10g carbohydrates, 1.4g fat, 3.1g fiber, 0mg cholesterol, 28mg sodium, 297mg potassium.

Zucchini Noodles Soup

Yield: 4 servings | **Prep time:** 10 minutes | **Cook time:** 15 minutes
- 2 zucchinis, trimmed
- 4 cups low-sodium chicken stock
- 2 oz fresh parsley, chopped
- ½ teaspoon chili flakes
- 1 oz carrot, shredded
- 1 teaspoon canola oil

1. Roast the carrot with canola oil in the saucepan for 5 minutes over the medium-low heat.
2. Stir it well and add chicken stock. Bring the mixture to boil.
3. Meanwhile, make the noodles from the zucchini with the help of the spiralizer.
4. Add them in the boiling soup liquid.
5. Add parsley and chili flakes. Bring the soup to boil and remove it from the heat.
6. Leave for 10 minutes to rest.

per serving: 39 calories, 2.7g protein, 4.9g carbohydrates, 1.5g fat, 1.7g fiber, 0mg cholesterol, 158mg sodium, 359mg potassium.

Grilled Tomatoes Soup

Yield: 4 servings | **Prep time:** 10 minutes | **Cook time:** 20 minutes
- 2-pounds tomatoes
- ½ cup shallot, chopped
- 1 tablespoon avocado oil
- ½ teaspoon ground black pepper
- ¼ teaspoon minced garlic
- 1 tablespoon dried basil
- 3 cups low-sodium chicken broth

1. Cut the tomatoes into halves and grill them in the preheated to 390F grill for 1 minute from each side.
2. After this, transfer the grilled tomatoes in the blender and blend until smooth.
3. Place the shallot and avocado oil in the saucepan and roast it until light brown.
4. Add blended grilled tomatoes, ground black pepper, and minced garlic.
5. Bring the soup to boil and sprinkle with dried basil.
6. Simmer the soup for 2 minutes more.

per serving: 72 calories, 4.1g protein, 13.4g carbohydrates, 0.9g fat, 3g fiber, 0mg cholesterol, 98mg sodium, 623mg potassium.

Chicken Oatmeal Soup

Yield: 5 servings | **Prep time:** 10 minutes | **Cook time:** 15 minutes
- 1 cup oats
- 4 cups of water
- 1 oz fresh dill, chopped
- 10 oz chicken fillet, chopped
- 1 teaspoon ground black pepper
- 1 teaspoon potato starch
- ½ carrot, diced

1. Put the chopped chicken in the saucepan, add water and bring it to boil. Simmer the chicken for 10 minutes.
2. Add dill, ground black pepper, oats, and diced carrot.
3. Bring the soup to boil and add potato starch. Stir it until soup starts to thicken. Simmer the soup for 5 minutes on the low heat.

per serving: 192 calories, 19.8g protein, 16.1g carbohydrates, 5.5g fat, 2.7g fiber, 50mg cholesterol, 72mg sodium, 411mg potassium.

Celery Cream Soup

Yield: 4 servings | **Prep time:** 10 minutes | **Cook time:** 25 minutes
- 2 cups celery stalk, chopped
- 1 shallot, chopped
- 1 potato, chopped
- 4 cups low-sodium vegetable stock
- 1 tablespoon margarine
- 1 teaspoon white pepper

1. Melt the margarine in the saucepan, add shallot, and celery stalk. Cook the vegetables for 5 minutes. Stir them occasionally.
2. After this, add vegetable stock and potato.
3. Simmer the soup for 15 minutes.
4. Blend the soup tilly ou get the creamy texture and sprinkle with white pepper.
5. Simmer it for 5 minutes more.

per serving: 88 calories, 2.3g protein, 13.3g carbohydrates, 3g fat, 2.9g fiber, 0mg cholesterol, 217mg sodium, 449mg potassium.

Cauliflower Soup

Yield: 2 servings | **Prep time:** 10 minutes | **Cook time:** 20 minutes
- 1 cup cauliflower, chopped
- ¼ cup potato, chopped
- 1 cup skim milk
- 1 cup of water
- 1 teaspoon ground coriander
- 1 teaspoon margarine

1. Put cauliflower and potato in the saucepan.
2. Add water and boil the ingredients for 15 minutes.
3. Then add ground coriander and margarine.
4. With the help of the immersion blender, blend the soup until smooth.
5. Add skim milk and stir well.

per serving: 82 calories, 5.2g protein, 10.3g carbohydrates, 2g fat, 1.5g fiber, 2mg cholesterol, 106mg sodium, 384mg potassium.

Buckwheat Soup

Yield: 6 servings | **Prep time:** 10 minutes | **Cook time:** 25 minutes
- ½ cup buckwheat
- 1 carrot, chopped
- 1 yellow onion, diced
- 1 tablespoon avocado oil
- 1 tablespoon fresh dill, chopped
- 1-pound chicken breast, chopped
- 1 teaspoon ground black pepper
- 6 cups of water

1. Saute the onion, carrot, and avocado oil in the saucepan for 5 minutes. Stir them from time to time.

2. Then add buckwheat, chicken breast, and ground black pepper.
3. Add water and close the lid.
4. Simmer the soup for 20 minutes.
5. After this, add dill and remove the soup from the heat. Leave it for 10 minutes to rest.

per serving: 152 calories, 18.4g protein, 13.5g carbohydrates, 2.7g fat, 2.3g fiber, 48mg cholesterol, 48mg sodium, 433mg potassium.

Parsley Soup

Yield: 6 servings | **Prep time:** 10 minutes | **Cook time:** 16 minutes

- 2 teaspoons olive oil
- 1 cup carrot, shredded
- 1 cup yellow onion, chopped
- 1 cup celery, chopped
- 6 cups of water
- 1 cup fresh parsley, chopped
- ¼ cup low-fat parmesan, grated

1. Heat up a pot with the oil over medium-high heat, add onion, carrot, and celery, stir and cook for 7 minutes.
2. Add water and all remaining ingredients.
3. Cook the soup for 8 minutes over the medium heat.

per serving: 46 calories, 1.6g protein, 4.8g carbohydrates, 2.5g fat, 1.5g fiber, 4mg cholesterol, 103mg sodium, 193mg potassium.

Tomato Bean Soup

Yield: 6 servings | **Prep time:** 10 minutes | **Cook time:** 25 minutes

- 2 teaspoons olive oil
- 2 garlic cloves, minced
- 1 pound green beans, trimmed and halved
- 4 tomatoes, cubed
- 1 teaspoon sweet paprika
- 4 cup of water
- 2 tablespoons dill, chopped

1. Heat up a pot with the oil over medium-high heat, add the garlic stir. Sauté the garlic for 5 minutes.
2. Add all remaining ingredients and cook the soup for 20 minutes.

per serving: 57 calories, 2.4g protein, 9.7g carbohydrates, 1.9g fat, 3.8g fiber, 0mg cholesterol, 16mg sodium, 400mg potassium.

Red Kidney Beans Soup

Yield: 4 servings | **Prep time:** 10 minutes | **Cook time:** 20 minutes

- 2 teaspoons olive oil
- 1 yellow onion, chopped
- 1 teaspoon cinnamon powder
- 1 cup red kidney beans, cooked
- 3 cups low-sodium chicken broth
- 1 potato, chopped

1. Heat up a pot with the oil over medium heat, add onion and cinnamon, stir and cook for 6 minutes.
2. Add all remaining ingredients and cook them for 14 minutes.
3. Blend the soup until you get puree texture.

per serving: 230 calories, 13g protein, 38.9g carbohydrates, 2.9g fat, 8.5g fiber, 0mg cholesterol, 62mg sodium, 844mg potassium.

Pork Soup

Yield: 4 servings | **Prep time:** 10 minutes | **Cook time:** 25 minutes

- 1 tablespoon avocado oil
- 1 onion, chopped
- 1 pound pork stew meat, cubed
- 4 cups of water
- 1 pound carrots, sliced
- 1 teaspoon tomato paste

1. Heat up a pot with the oil over medium-high heat, add the onion and pork, and cook the ingredients for 5 minutes.
2. Add all remaining ingredients and cook the soup for 20 minutes.

per serving: 304 calories, 34.5g protein, 14.2g carbohydrates, 11.4g fat, 3.6g fiber, 98mg cholesterol, 155mg sodium, 855mg potassium.

Curry Soup

Yield: 4 servings | **Prep time:** 10 minutes | **Cook time:** 23 minutes

- 3 tablespoons olive oil
- 8 carrots, peeled and sliced
- 2 teaspoons curry paste
- 4 celery stalks, chopped
- 1 yellow onion, chopped

- *4 cups of water*

1. Heat up a pot with the oil and add onion, celery and carrots, stir and cook for 12 minutes.
2. Then add curry paste and water. Stir the soup well and cook it for 10 minutes more.
3. When all ingredients are soft, blend the soup until smooth and simmer it for 1 minute more.

per serving: 171 calories, 1.6g protein, 15.8g carbohydrates, 12g fat, 3.9g fiber, 0mg cholesterol, 106mg sodium, 477mg potassium.

Yellow Onion Soup

Yield: 4 servings | **Prep time:** 10 minutes | **Cook time:** 20 minutes

- *1 tablespoon avocado oil*
- *1 yellow onion, chopped*
- *1 teaspoon ginger, grated*
- *1 pound zucchinis, chopped*
- *4 cups low-sodium chicken broth*
- *½ cup low-fat cream*
- *1 teaspoon ground black pepper*

1. Heat up a pot with the oil over medium heat, add the onion and ginger, stir and cook for 5 minutes.
2. Add all remaining ingredients and simmer them over medium heat for 15 minutes.
3. Blend the cooked soup and ladle in the bowls.

per serving: 61 calories, 4.2g protein, 10.2g carbohydrates, 0.7g fat, 2.2g fiber, 1mg cholesterol, 101mg sodium, 377mg potassium.

Garlic Soup

Yield: 4 servings | **Prep time:** 10 minutes | **Cook time:** 50 minutes

- *1 pound red kidney beans, cooked*
- *8 cups of water*
- *1 green bell pepper, chopped*
- *1 tomato paste*
- *1 yellow onion, chopped*
- *1 teaspoon minced garlic*
- *1 pound beef sirloin, cubed*
- *1 teaspoon garlic powder*

1. Pour water in a pot and heat up over medium heat.
2. Add all ingredients and close the lid.
3. Simmer the soup for 45 minutes over the medium heat.

per serving: 620 calories, 60.9g protein, 75.8g carbohydrates, 8.4g fat, 18.5g fiber, 101mg cholesterol, 109mg sodium, 2150mg potassium.

Poultry Soup

Yield: 4 servings | **Prep time:** 10 minutes | **Cook time:** 40 minutes

- *3 oz turkey breast, skinless, boneless, chopped*
- *1 tablespoon tomato paste*
- *1 tablespoon olive oil*
- *2 yellow onions, chopped*
- *4 cups of water*
- *1 tablespoon oregano, chopped*
- *¼ cup carrot, diced*

1. Heat up a pot with the oil over medium heat, add the onions and sauté for 5 minutes.
2. Add the turkey and brown it for 5 minutes more.
3. Add the rest of the ingredients, bring to a simmer and cook over medium heat for 30 minutes.

per serving: 84 calories, 4.6g protein, 8.2g carbohydrates, 4.1g fat, 2.1g fiber, 9mg cholesterol, 236mg sodium, 229mg potassium.

Roasted Tomatoes Soup

Yield: 4 servings | **Prep time:** 10 minutes | **Cook time:** 20 minutes

- *1 yellow onion, chopped*
- *1 carrot, chopped*
- *1 tablespoon olive oil*
- *15 ounces roasted tomatoes, no-salt-added*
- *2 cups of water*
- *1 tablespoon tomato paste*
- *1 tablespoon basil, dried*
- *¼ teaspoon oregano, dried*
- *1 teaspoon chili powder*

1. Heat up a pot with the oil over medium heat, add onion, stir and cook for 5 minutes.
2. Add all remaining ingredients and simmer them for 15 minutes.

3. Then blend the soup until you get the creamy texture.
per serving: 78 calories, 1.5g protein, 9.4g carbohydrates, 3.7g fat, 2.2g fiber, 0mg cholesterol, 38mg sodium, 147mg potassium.

Yogurt Soup

Yield: 4 servings | **Prep time:** 10 minutes | **Cook time:** 20 minutes
- 3 garlic cloves, minced
- 1 onion, chopped
- 3 carrots, chopped
- 1 tablespoon olive oil
- 2 cups tomatillos, chopped
- 2 cups low-sodium chicken broth
- ½ cup low-fat yogurt
- 1 teaspoon white pepper

1. Heat up a pot with the oil over medium heat, add the onion and the garlic and sauté for 5 minutes.
2. Add all the remaining ingredients and cook the soup for 15 minutes more.
per serving: 152 calories, 18.4g protein, 13.5g carbohydrates, 2.7g fat, 2.3g fiber, 48mg cholesterol, 48mg sodium, 433mg potassium.

Fish Soup

Yield: 4 servings | **Prep time:** 10 minutes | **Cook time:** 25 minutes
- 1 yellow onion, chopped
- 4 cups of water
- 1 teaspoon ground coriander
- 2 tablespoons fresh dill, chopped
- 1 teaspoon ground black pepper
- 1 tablespoon avocado oil
- 1 pound cod, skinless, boneless and cut into medium chunks

1. Heat up a pot with the oil over medium-high heat, add onion, stir and cook for 4 minutes.
2. Add all remaining ingredients and cook the soup for 20 minutes over the medium heat.
per serving: 140 calories, 26.6g protein, 4g carbohydrates, 1.5g fat, 1.1g fiber, 62mg cholesterol, 100mg sodium, 389mg potassium.

Trout Soup

Yield: 4 servings | **Prep time:** 10 minutes | **Cook time:** 25 minutes
- 4 cups of water
- 1 pound trout fillets, boneless, skinless and cubed
- 1 tablespoon sweet paprika
- 1 tablespoon olive oil
- 1 bell pepper, chopped
- 2 oz celery stalk, chopped

1. Heat up a pot with the oil over medium-high heat, add the celery stalk, stir and sauté for 5 minutes.
2. Add the fish and all remaining ingredients and simmer the soup over medium heat for 20 minutes.
per serving: 262 calories, 32.9g protein, 3.6g carbohydrates, 13.4g fat, 1.3g fiber, 84mg cholesterol, 96mg sodium, 661mg potassium.

Nutmeg Soup

Yield: 6 servings | **Prep time:** 10 minutes | **Cook time:** 60 minutes
- 2 cups sweet potatoes
- 5 cups of water
- 1 teaspoon nutmeg, ground
- 1 cup low-fat yogurt

1. Arrange the sweet potatoes on a lined baking sheet, bake them at 350F for 40 minutes, cool them down, peel, roughly chop them and put them in a pot.
2. Add all remaining ingredients and cook the soup for 20 minutes.
per serving: 90 calories, 3.1g protein, 17g carbohydrates, 0.7g fat, 2.1g fiber, 2mg cholesterol, 39mg sodium, 507mg potassium.

Quinoa Soup

Yield: 6 servings | **Prep time:** 10 minutes | **Cook time:** 60 minutes
- 2 pounds chicken breast, skinless and boneless and cubed
- 2 red bell peppers, chopped
- 1 tablespoon olive oil
- 2 cups quinoa, already cooked
- ¼ cup cilantro, chopped
- 2 tablespoons lemon juice
- ½ teaspoon ground black pepper
- 4 cups of water
- 1 cup low-fat milk

1. Heat up a pot with the oil over medium-high heat, add chicken and cook it for 5 minutes on each side.
2. Add all remaining ingredients except quinoa and cook the soup for 40 minutes.
3. Then add quinoa, stir it well and cook for 15 minutes more.

per serving: 433 calories, 41.9g protein, 41.7g carbohydrates, 10.1g fat, 4.6g fiber, 99mg cholesterol, 105mg sodium, 1028mg potassium.

Red Eggplant Soup

Yield: 4 servings | **Prep time:** 10 minutes | **Cook time:** 30 minutes
- 2 big eggplants, roughly cubed
- 4 cups of water
- 2 tablespoons tomato paste
- 1 tablespoon olive oil
- 2 tablespoons parsley, chopped
- 1 teaspoon ground turmeric

1. Heat up a pot with the oil over medium heat, add eggplants and sauté them for 5 minutes.
2. Add all remaining ingredients and cook the soup for 25 minutes more.

per serving: 108 calories, 3.1g protein, 18.1g carbohydrates, 4.1g fat, 10.2g fiber, 0mg cholesterol, 22mg sodium, 735mg potassium.

Milk Soup

Yield: 8 servings | **Prep time:** 10 minutes | **Cook time:** 20 minutes
- 4 cups low-fat milk
- 2 tablespoons olive oil
- 2 sweet potatoes, peeled and cubed
- 2 yellow onions, chopped
- 2 cups of water
- 1 teaspoon ground black pepper
- 4 tablespoons dill, chopped
- ½ teaspoon basil, chopped

1. Heat up a pot with the oil over medium heat, add onion, stir and cook for 5 minutes.
2. Add all remaining ingredients and simmer the soup for 15 minutes.
3. Then blend the soup till you get a creamy texture.
4. The soups are cooked.

per serving: 97 calories, 4.8g protein, 9.8g carbohydrates, 4.8g fat, 0.9g fiber, 6mg cholesterol, 60mg sodium, 281mg potassium.

White Mushrooms Soup

Yield: 4 servings | **Prep time:** 10 minutes | **Cook time:** 30 minutes
- 4 cups of water
- 1 yellow onion, chopped
- 1 tablespoon olive oil
- 8 oz chicken breast, skinless, boneless, chopped
- ½ pound white mushrooms, chopped
- 1 chili pepper, chopped
- 2 tablespoons low-fat yogurt

1. Heat up a pot with the oil over medium heat, add the onion, chilies, chicken breast, and mushrooms and cook the ingredients for 10 minutes.
2. Add all remaining ingredients and cook the soup for 20 minutes. Let the cooked soup rest for 10 minutes before serving.

per serving: 124 calories, 14.6g protein, 5.1g carbohydrates, 5.2g fat, 1.2g fiber, 37mg cholesterol, 46mg sodium, 453mg potassium.

Cheese Soup with Cauliflower

Yield: 4 servings | **Prep time:** 10 minutes | **Cook time:** 45 minutes
- 3 pounds cauliflower, chopped
- 2 cups of water
- 1 cup low-fat yogurt
- 3 oz low-fat goat cheese, crumbled
- 1 teaspoon ground black pepper
- 2 tablespoons parsley, chopped

1. Put all ingredients in the saucepan.
2. Bring the soup to boil and cook for 35 minutes.
3. Then blend the soup with the help of the immersion blender and cook for 10 minutes more.

per serving: 227 calories, 16.8g protein, 23.3g carbohydrates, 8.7g fat, 8.7g fiber, 26mg cholesterol, 223mg sodium, 1203mg potassium.

Chicken-Asparagus Soup

Yield: 6 servings | **Prep time:** 10 minutes | **Cook time:** 30 minutes
- 12 oz chicken breasts, cooked, shredded

- *1 tablespoon olive oil*
- *½ teaspoon chili flakes*
- *1 yellow onion, finely chopped*
- *8 oz asparagus*
- *1 tablespoon lemon juice*
- *1 cup low-fat yogurt*
- *4 cups of water*

1. Heat up a pot with the oil over medium heat, add onions, stir and cook for 5 minutes.
2. Add asparagus, stir and cook for 5 minutes.
3. Add all remaining ingredients and cook the soup for 20 minutes over the medium heat.

per serving: 172 calories, 19.8g protein, 6.1g carbohydrates, 7.1g fat, 1.2g fiber, 53mg cholesterol, 84mg sodium, 341mg potassium.

Red Cabbage Soup

Yield: 4 servings | **Prep time:** 10 minutes | **Cook time:** 40 minutes

- *1-pound red cabbage, shredded*
- *1 yellow onion, chopped*
- *1 tablespoon olive oil*
- *1 teaspoon dried oregano*
- *3 oz leek, chopped*
- *3 cups low-sodium chicken broth*

1. Heat up a pot with the oil over medium heat, add the onion and the leek, stir and cook for 5 minutes.
2. Add the cabbage and all remaining ingredients from the list above and cook over medium heat for 35 minutes.

per serving: 95 calories, 3.6g protein, 13.2g carbohydrates, 3.7g fat, 4g fiber, 0mg cholesterol, 78mg sodium, 278mg potassium.

Celery and Leek Soup

Yield: 4 servings | **Prep time:** 10 minutes | **Cook time:** 60 minutes

- *2 cups celery stalk, chopped*
- *1 yellow onion, chopped*
- *1 tablespoon olive oil*
- *1 teaspoon chili flakes*
- *1 cup leek, chopped*
- *3 cups low-sodium chicken broth*
- *½ teaspoon dried sage*

1. Heat up a pot with the oil over medium-high heat, add the onion, celery, and leek, stir and cook for 5 minutes.
2. Add remaining ingredients and cook the soup for 55 minutes.
3. Blend the cooked soup with the immersion blender until smooth.

per serving: 74 calories, 2.5g protein, 8.1g carbohydrates, 3.7g fat, 1.8g fiber, 0mg cholesterol, 99mg sodium, 213mg potassium.

Collard Greens Soup

Yield: 4 servings | **Prep time:** 10 minutes | **Cook time:** 30 minutes

- *4 cups low-sodium chicken broth*
- *8 ounces chicken breast, skinless, boneless and chopped*
- *2 cups collard greens, chopped*
- *½ teaspoon dried oregano*
- *½ teaspoon white pepper*
- *½ teaspoon ground paprika*

1. Put the broth in a pot, chicken, oregano, white pepper, and ground paprika. Boil the ingredients over medium heat for 20 minutes.
2. Add collard greens and cook it for 10 more minutes.

per serving: 88 calories, 14.6g protein, 2.7g carbohydrates, 1.6g fat, 1g fiber, 36mg cholesterol, 103mg sodium, 222mg potassium.

Stalk Soup

Yield: 4 servings | **Prep time:** 10 minutes | **Cook time:** 40 minutes

- *2 pounds cauliflower florets*
- *1 tablespoon olive oil*
- *1 cup tomato puree*
- *1 cup celery, chopped*
- *6 cups low-sodium chicken broth*
- *3 tablespoons fresh cilantro, chopped*
- *1 teaspoon curry powder*

1. Heat up a pot with the oil over medium-high heat, add the celery, stir and sauté for 5 minutes.
2. After this, add all remaining ingredients and simmer the soup for 35 minutes.

per serving: 139 calories, 8.8g protein, 20.2g carbohydrates, 4g fat, 7.5g fiber, 0mg cholesterol, 211mg sodium, 1039mg potassium.

Cauliflower-Potato Soup

Yield: 6 servings | **Prep time:** 10 minutes | **Cook time:** 40 minutes
- 2 russet potatoes, chopped
- 1 cup cauliflower florets
- 5 cups low-sodium chicken broth
- ½ cup low-fat yogurt
- 1 teaspoon ground paprika
- 1 teaspoon chili powder
- 1 teaspoon dried oregano

1. Heat up a pot with the oil over medium-high heat, add cauliflower and potato, stir and cook for 5 minutes.
2. Add all remaining ingredients and cook the soup over medium heat for 30 minutes, blend using an immersion blender and simmer the soup for 2 minutes.

per serving: 83 calories, 4.5g protein, 14.9g carbohydrates, 0.5g fat, 2.5g fiber, 1mg cholesterol, 86mg sodium, 408mg potassium.

Green Chicken Soup

Yield: 4 servings | **Prep time:** 15 minutes | **Cook time:** 60 minutes
- 1-pound chicken breast, chopped
- ½ teaspoon ground black pepper
- 4 cups of water
- 1 cup spinach, chopped
- 2 cups yellow onion, chopped
- 1 teaspoon dried cilantro

1. Put the chicken in a pot, add the water and ingredients from the list above except spinach.
2. Cook the soup for 50 minutes.
3. Then add spinach and simmer the soup over the low heat for 10 minutes more.

per serving: 155 calories, 24.9g protein, 5.8g carbohydrates, 2.9g fat, 1.5g fiber, 73mg cholesterol, 73mg sodium, 551mg potassium.

Coriander Seafood Soup

Yield: 4 servings | **Prep time:** 10 minutes | **Cook time:** 20 minutes
- 4 cups of water
- ½ pound shrimp, peeled
- ½ pound cod fillets, chopped
- 2 tablespoons olive oil
- 1 teaspoon ground coriander
- 1 teaspoon smoked paprika
- 1 shallot, diced

1. Heat up a pot with the oil over medium heat, add the shallots, stir and sauté for 5 minutes.
2. Add the shrimp and the cod, and cook for 5 minutes more.
3. After this, add the ground coriander and smoked paprika. Stir the soup and cook it for 10 minutes more over the medium heat.

per serving: 178 calories, 23.2g protein, 2g carbohydrates, 8.6g fat, 0.2g fiber, 147mg cholesterol, 182mg sodium, 128mg potassium.

Chicken Broth and Shrimps Soup

Yield: 6 servings | **Prep time:** 10 minutes | **Cook time:** 15 minutes
- 6 cups low-sodium chicken broth
- 3 cups shrimp, peeled and deveined
- 3 oz scallions, chopped
- 2 tablespoons chives, chopped

1. Put all ingredients in the saucepan and bring to boil.
2. Simmer the soup for 10 minutes over the medium heat.

per serving: 50 calories, 8.8g protein, 2.1g carbohydrates, 0.2g fat, 0.4g fiber, 123mg cholesterol, 287mg sodium, 42mg potassium.

Chili Pepper Soup

Yield: 4 servings | **Prep time:** 5 minutes | **Cook time:** 30 minutes
- ½ cup millet
- 1 carrot, chopped
- 1 yellow onion, diced
- 5 cups of water
- 1 chili pepper, chopped
- 1 tablespoon margarine

1. Heat up a pot with the oil, over medium heat, add the onion, chili pepper, margarine, and carrot. Cook the ingredients for 5 minutes.
2. Then add millet and water, and stir the soup well.

per serving: 138 calories, 3.2g protein, 22.4g carbohydrates, 3.9g fat, 3.1g fiber, 0mg cholesterol, 55mg sodium, 145mg potassium.

Kale and Mushrooms Soup

Yield: 4 servings | **Prep time:** 10 minutes | **Cook time:** 25 minutes
- 1 yellow onion, chopped

- *½ teaspoon white pepper*
- *1 tablespoon olive oil*
- *½ teaspoon cayenne pepper*
- *2 cups kale, chopped*
- *1 cup cremini mushrooms, chopped*
- *4 cups low-sodium chicken broth*

1. Heat up olive oil in the saucepan.
2. Add onion, white pepper, cayenne pepper, and mushrooms. Cook the ingredients for 5 minutes.
3. Then add chicken broth and kale.
4. Cook the soup for 15 minutes.

per serving: 79 calories, 3.8g protein, 8.1g carbohydrates, 3.6g fat, 1.3g fiber, 0mg cholesterol, 87mg sodium, 293mg potassium.

Chicken and Sweet Potato Aromatic Soup

Yield: 6 servings | **Prep time:** 10 minutes | **Cook time:** 20 minutes

- *1-pound chicken breast, skinless, boneless, chopped*
- *1 onion, chopped*
- *2 tablespoons olive oil*
- *1 cup sweet potatoes, cubed*
- *A pinch of black pepper*
- *5 cups low-sodium chicken broth*

1. Roast the chicken breast with olive oil in the saucepan for 5 minutes.
2. Then add all remaining ingredients from the list above and cook them on the medium heat for 15 minutes.
3. Let the cooked soup rest for 10 minutes before serving.

per serving: 192 calories, 20.8g protein, 8.7g carbohydrates, 7.8g fat, 1.4g fiber, 48mg cholesterol, 150mg sodium, 511mg potassium.

Salads

Salad Skewers

Yield: 4 servings | **Prep time:** 10 minutes | **Cook time:** 0 minutes

- 2 cucumbers
- 2 cups cherry tomatoes
- ½ teaspoon lemon juice
- 1 teaspoon olive oil

1. Cut the cucumbers on medium cubes.
2. Then string the cucumber cubes and cherry tomatoes into skewers one-by-one.
3. Then sprinkle the salad skewers with lemon juice and olive oil.

per serving: 49 calories, 1.8g protein, 9g carbohydrates, 1.5g fat, 1.8g fiber, 0mg cholesterol, 8mg sodium, 435mg potassium.

Nectarine Salad with Shrimps

Yield: 4 servings | **Prep time:** 7 minutes | **Cook time:** 6 minutes

- 1 cup spring mix salad greens
- 1 nectarine, pitted, chopped
- 6 oz shrimps, peeled
- 1 tablespoon olive oil
- 1 teaspoon lemon juice
- ¼ teaspoon ground black pepper
- 1 teaspoon margarine

1. Toss the margarine in the skillet and melt it.
2. Mix up ground black pepper and shrimps.
3. Then place the shrimps in the hot margarine and cook for 3 minutes from each side.
4. Transfer the cooked shrimps in the salad bowl.
5. Add spring mix salad greens, chopped nectarine, olive oil, and lemon juice.
6. Shake the salad.

per serving: 110 calories, 10.6g protein, 4.5g carbohydrates, 5.4g fat, 0.9g fiber, 90mg cholesterol, 125mg sodium, 98mg potassium.

Asian Style Cobb Salad

Yield: 4 servings | **Prep time:** 10 minutes | **Cook time:** 0 minutes

- 2 cup lettuce, chopped
- 1 cup tangerines, peeled
- 1 cup carrot, grated
- 3 oz scallions, chopped
- 1 avocado, sliced
- 3 tablespoons balsamic vinegar
- 1 tablespoon sesame seeds
- 1 tablespoon lemon zest, grated
- 1 tablespoon avocado oil

1. Make the salad dressing: mix up balsamic vinegar, sesame seeds, lemon zest, and avocado oil.
2. Put all remaining ingredients in the bowl and sprinkle with salad dressing.
3. Shake the salad gently before serving.

per serving: 195 calories, 2.5g protein, 16.3g carbohydrates, 14.5g fat, 5.6g fiber, 0mg cholesterol, 31mg sodium, 535mg potassium.

Tomato Salad

Yield: 2 servings | **Prep time:** 10 minutes | **Cook time:** 0 minutes
- 1 red onion, sliced
- 2 cups cherry tomatoes, halved
- ¼ teaspoon ground black pepper
- ½ cup fresh cilantro, chopped
- 1 tablespoon olive oil
- ½ teaspoon dried oregano
- 1 tablespoon apple cider vinegar

1. Mix up cherry tomatoes and sliced red onion.
2. Add cilantro. Mix up the salad.
3. After this, sprinkle the salad with ground black pepper, olive oil, dried oregano, apple cider vinegar.
4. Shake the salad gently.

per serving: 119 calories, 2.4g protein, 12.8g carbohydrates, 7.5g fat, 3.7g fiber, 0mg cholesterol, 13mg sodium, 543mg potassium.

Cheese&Steak Salad

Yield: 7 servings | **Prep time:** 10 minutes | **Cook time:** 18 minutes
- 10 oz beef sirloin steak
- 1 teaspoon beef seasonings
- 3 cups Romaine lettuce, chopped
- 1 cup sweet pepper, chopped
- 7 oz low-fat cheese, crumbled
- 1 cup cucumbers, chopped
- 1 tablespoon olive oil
- 1 teaspoon avocado oil
- 1 teaspoon balsamic vinegar

1. Rub the beef sirloin steak with beef seasonings and avocado oil.
2. Preheat the grill to 400F and put the steak in it.
3. Cook it for 9 minutes from each side.
4. When the steak is cooked, slice it and put it in the salad bowl.
5. Add romaine lettuce, sweet pepper, cucumbers, and shake well.
6. Sprinkle the salad with olive oil and balsamic vinegar.
7. Then top the salad with crumbled cheese.

per serving: 219 calories, 19.7g protein, 3g carbohydrates, 14.1g fat, 0.5g fiber, 66mg cholesterol, 205mg sodium, 281mg potassium.

Corn Salad with Spinach

Yield: 3 servings | **Prep time:** 5 minutes | **Cook time:** 0 minutes
- 1 cup corn kernels, cooked
- 1 teaspoon low-fat sour cream
- 1 cup fresh spinach, chopped
- ½ cup celery stalk, chopped

1. Mix up corn kernels, spinach, and celery stalk in the salad bowl.
2. Then sprinkle the cooked salad with low-fat sour cream.

per serving: 52 calories, 2.1g protein, 10.6g carbohydrates, 1g fat, 1.9g fiber, 1mg cholesterol, 30mg sodium, 240mg potassium.

Shredded Beef Salad

Yield: 4 servings | **Prep time:** 10 minutes | **Cook time:** 0 minutes
- 8 oz beef sirloin, cooked, shredded
- 1 tablespoon mustard
- 1 bell pepper, sliced
- 2 cups lettuce, chopped
- 1 teaspoon lime juice

1. In the salad bowl mix up bell pepper, lettuce, and shredded beef sirloin.
2. Sprinkle the salad with lime juice and mustard. Shake it.

per serving: 133 calories, 18.3g protein, 4.3g carbohydrates, 4.5g fat, 1g fiber, 51mg cholesterol, 40mg sodium, 345mg potassium.

Tangerine and Edamame Salad

Yield: 4 servings | **Prep time:** 10 minutes | **Cook time:** 10 minutes
- ½ cup edamame beans, soaked
- 2 cups of water
- 1 cup corn kernels, cooked
- ½ cup Italian parsley, chopped
- 1 tablespoon olive oil
- 1 teaspoon chili flakes
- ½ teaspoon ground black pepper
- 1 cup tangerines, peeled

1. Pour water in the saucepan. Add edamame beans and boil them for 10 minutes.
2. After this, drain and rinse the edamame beans and transfer them in the salad bowl.
3. Add cooked corn kernels, parsley, and tangerines.

4.   Then sprinkle the salad with ground black pepper, chili flakes, and olive oil.
5.   Stir the salad.
per serving: 113 calories, 4g protein, 15.8g carbohydrates, 5g fat, 2.8g fiber, 0mg cholesterol, 17mg sodium, 234mg potassium.

Chicken Salad in Jars

Yield: 4 servings | **Prep time:** 10 minutes | **Cook time:** 0 minutes
- 1 cup apples, chopped
- ½ cup grapes, halved
- 1 cup lettuce, chopped
- 1-pound chicken breast, boiled, chopped
- ¼ cup low-fat Greek yogurt
- ½ teaspoon ground black pepper
- ¼ teaspoon ground paprika
- 1 teaspoon lemon juice

1.   Make the dressing: mix up lemon juice, ground paprika, ground black pepper, and Greek yogurt.
2.   Then pour the dressing in jars.
3.   Add the layer of apples, then lettuce, chicken, and grapes.
4.   Top the salad jars with remaining yogurt dressing.
per serving: 184 calories, 25g protein, 13.2g carbohydrates, 3.2g fat, 1.7g fiber, 73mg cholesterol, 68mg sodium, 556mg potassium.

Farro Salad

Yield: 3 servings | **Prep time:** 10 minutes | **Cook time:** 30 minutes
- 1 cup arugula, chopped
- 3 oz walnuts, chopped
- 1 apple, chopped
- 1 cup of water
- ½ cup farro
- 1 teaspoon honey
- 1 tablespoon low-fat sour cream
- ¼ teaspoon chili powder

1.   Mix up water and farro.
2.   Cook the farro for 30 minutes.
3.   Then drain the remaining water and place the farro in the bowl.
4.   Add walnuts, apple, arugula, and mix up the salad.
5.   After this, in the shallow bowl, mix up honey, low-fat sour cream, and chili powder.
6.   Sprinkle the salad with honey mixture.
per serving: 339 calories, 12g protein, 37.5g carbohydrates, 17.8g fat, 5.9g fiber, 2mg cholesterol, 30mg sodium, 264mg potassium.

Warm Lentil Salad

Yield: 6 servings | **Prep time:** 10 minutes | **Cook time:** 15 minutes
- 1 cup green lentils
- 2 cups low-sodium chicken broth
- 1 yellow onion, sliced
- ½ teaspoon dried sage
- 2 tablespoons olive oil
- 1 cup celery stalk, chopped
- 6 oz swiss chard, steamed, chopped
- ½ teaspoon cayenne pepper

1.   Boil lentils in the chicken broth. Boil it for 15 minutes.
2.   After this, transfer the cooked lentils in the salad bowl.
3.   Add 1 tablespoon of olive oil.
4.   Pour the remaining olive oil in the skillet.
5.   Add sliced yellow onion and cook it until golden brown.
6.   Add the cooked onion in the lentils.
7.   Then add celery stalk, swiss chard, sage, and cayenne pepper. Stir the salad.
per serving: 174 calories, 9.8g protein, 23g carbohydrates, 5.2g fat, 11g fiber, 0mg cholesterol, 100mg sodium, 487mg potassium.

Grilled Cod and Blue Cheese Salad

Yield: 4 servings | **Prep time:** 10 minutes | **Cook time:** 8 minutes
- 1 cup arugula, chopped
- 12 oz cod fillet
- ½ teaspoon ground coriander
- 1 teaspoon apple cider vinegar
- 1 teaspoon olive oil
- 1 tablespoon sesame oil
- ½ teaspoon sesame seeds
- 1 oz blue cheese, crumbled

1.   Preheat the grill to 390F.
2.   Meanwhile, sprinkle the cod fillet with apple cider vinegar, ground coriander, and olive oil.
3.   Put the fish fillets in the grill and cook for 4 minutes from each side.
4.   Meanwhile, in the salad bowl, mix up chopped arugula, sesame seeds, blue cheese, and sesame oil.

5. When the fish is cooked, chop it roughly and add in the salad. Shake it well.
per serving: 91 calories, 6.7g protein, 0.5g carbohydrates, 7g fat, 0.1g fiber, 20mg cholesterol, 114mg sodium, 21mg potassium.

Tabbouleh Salad

Yield: 4 servings | **Prep time:** 10 minutes | **Cook time:** 15 minutes
- ¼ cup bulgur
- 7 oz cucumber, diced
- 3 tomatoes, diced
- ½ cup dill, chopped
- 3 oz scallions, chopped
- ½ teaspoon garlic, diced
- 1 cup of water
- ½ teaspoon chili powder

1. Boil the bulgur in water for 15 minutes.
2. Then transfer the cooked bulgur in the bowl.
3. Add diced cucumber, tomato, dill, scallions, garlic, and chili powder.
4. Carefully stir the salad.

per serving: 78 calories, 3.9g protein, 17.2g carbohydrates, 0.7g fat, 4.5g fiber, 0mg cholesterol, 28mg sodium, 593mg potassium.

Fattoush

Yield: 2 servings | **Prep time:** 10 minutes | **Cook time:** 0 minutes
- ½ teaspoon sumac
- 1 cup lettuce leaves, chopped
- 1 cup cucumbers, chopped
- 1 cup tomatoes, chopped
- 1 tablespoon fresh mint, chopped
- 2 oz white onion, sliced
- 1 garlic clove, minced
- 2 tablespoons lime juice
- 1 tablespoon apple cider vinegar
- 1 teaspoon olive oil

1. For the dressing: mix up minced garlic, lime juice, apple cider vinegar, and sumac. Whisk it.
2. In the salad bowl, mix up lettuce, cucumbers, tomatoes, fresh mint, and white onion.
3. Sprinkle the salad ingredients with dressing and shake well.

per serving: 67 calories, 1.8g protein, 10.7g carbohydrates, 2.7g fat, 2.4g fiber, 0mg cholesterol, 12mg sodium, 406mg potassium.

Couscous Salad

Yield: 5 servings | **Prep time:** 10 minutes | **Cook time:** 5 minutes
- ½ cup couscous
- 1 cup hot water
- ½ cup chickpeas, canned
- 1 teaspoon olive oil
- ½ teaspoon ground cumin
- 2 cups arugula, chopped
- ¼ cup red onion, chopped
- 3 tablespoon lemon juice
- 3 oz sun-dried tomatoes, sliced

1. Put couscous and chickpeas in the big bowl.
2. Add hot water and mix the mixture up. Leave it for 5 minutes.
3. After this, add olive oil, ground cumin, arugula, red onion, lemon juice, and sun-dried tomatoes.
4. Mix up the salad well.

per serving: 156 calories, 6.6g protein, 27.3g carbohydrates, 2.5g fat, 4.9g fiber, 0mg cholesterol, 13mg sodium, 298mg potassium.

Celeriac Salad

Yield: 4 servings | **Prep time:** 5 minutes | **Cook time:** 0 minutes
- 1 cup carrot, shredded
- 1 cup celery root, grated
- 1 oz raisins
- ½ cup apples, grated
- 1 teaspoon olive oil
- 1 teaspoon liquid honey

1. Mix up carrot, celery root, raisins, and apples.
2. Then mix up olive oil and liquid honey.
3. Sprinkle the salad with the oily mixture.

per serving: 79 calories, 1.1g protein, 17.2g carbohydrates, 1.4g fat, 2.3g fiber, 0mg cholesterol, 59mg sodium, 289mg potassium.

Crunchy Lettuce Salad

Yield: 3 servings | **Prep time:** 5 minutes | **Cook time:** 0 minutes
- 2 cups lettuce, chopped
- 1 cup cucumbers, chopped
- ½ cup fresh dill, chopped
- 1 orange, peeled, sliced
- 1 tablespoon olive oil

- 1 teaspoon apple cider vinegar
1. In the salad bowl, mix up lettuce, cucumbers, dill, and sprinkle with olive oil and apple cider vinegar.
2. Top the salad with sliced orange.

per serving: 100 calories, 2.6g protein, 14.1g carbohydrates, 5.2g fat, 3g fiber, 0mg cholesterol, 19mg sodium, 480mg potassium.

Herbed Melon Salad

Yield: 5 servings | **Prep time:** 5 minutes | **Cook time:** 0 minutes
- 2 cups melon, chopped
- ¼ cup grapes, chopped
- 1 cup cucumbers, chopped
- 3 oz low-fat feta cheese, chopped
- 1 teaspoon Italian seasonings
- ¼ teaspoon ground black pepper
- ¼ cup of orange juice
- 1 tablespoon avocado oil

1. Mix up melon, grapes, cucumbers, Italian seasonings, and ground black pepper.
2. Then add orange juice and avocado oil. Stir the salad well.
3. Sprinkle the cooked salad with chopped low-fat feta cheese.

per serving: 85 calories, 3.2g protein, 9g carbohydrates, 4.5g fat, 0.9g fiber, 16mg cholesterol, 201mg sodium, 252mg potassium.

Spring Greens Salad

Yield: 2 servings | **Prep time:** 5 minutes | **Cook time:** 0 minutes
- ½ cup radish, sliced
- 1 cup fresh spinach, chopped
- ½ cup green peas, cooked
- ½ lemon
- 1 cup arugula, chopped
- 1 tablespoon avocado oil
- ½ teaspoon dried sage

1. In the salad bowl, mix up radish, spinach, green peas, arugula, and dried sage.
2. Then squeeze the lemon over the salad.
3. Add avocado oil and shake the salad.

per serving: 54 calories, 3.1g protein, 9g carbohydrates, 1.3g fat, 3.6g fiber, 0mg cholesterol, 28mg sodium, 321mg potassium.

Tuna Salad

Yield: 4 servings | **Prep time:** 7 minutes | **Cook time:** 0 minutes
- ½ cup low-fat Greek yogurt
- 8 oz tuna, canned
- ½ cup fresh parsley, chopped
- 1 cup corn kernels, cooked
- ½ teaspoon ground black pepper

1. Mix up tuna, parsley, kernels, and ground black pepper.
2. Then add yogurt and stir the salad until it is homogenous.

per serving: 172 calories, 17.8g protein, 13.6g carbohydrates, 5.5g fat, 1.4g fiber, 19mg cholesterol, 55mg sodium, 392mg potassium.

Fish Salad

Yield: 4 servings | **Prep time:** 5 minutes | **Cook time:** 0 minutes
- 7 oz canned salmon, shredded
- 1 tablespoon lime juice
- 1 tablespoon low-fat yogurt
- 1 cup baby spinach, chopped
- 1 teaspoon capers, drained and chopped

1. Mix up all ingredients together and transfer them in the salad bowl.

per serving: 71 calories, 10.1g protein, 0.8g carbohydrates, 3.2g fat, 0.2g fiber, 22mg cholesterol, 52mg sodium, 244mg potassium.

Salmon Salad

Yield: 3 servings | **Prep time:** 10 minutes | **Cook time:** 0 minutes
- 4 oz canned salmon, flaked
- 1 tablespoon lemon juice
- 2 tablespoons red bell pepper, chopped
- 1 tablespoon red onion, chopped
- 1 teaspoon dill, chopped
- 1 tablespoon olive oil

1. Mix up all ingredients in the salad bowl.

per serving: 119 calories, 8.3g protein, 6.6g carbohydrates, 7.3g fat, 1.2g fiber, 17mg cholesterol, 21mg sodium, 317mg potassium.

Arugula Salad with Shallot

Yield: 4 servings | **Prep time:** 10 minutes | **Cook time:** 0 minutes
- 1 cup cucumber, chopped
- 1 tablespoon lemon juice

- 1 tablespoon avocado oil
- 2 shallots, chopped
- ½ cup black olives, sliced
- 3 cups arugula, chopped

1. Mix up all ingredients from the list above in the salad bowl and refrigerate in the fridge for 5 minutes.

per serving: 33 calories, 0.8g protein, 2.9g carbohydrates, 2.4g fat, 1.1g fiber, 0mg cholesterol, 152mg sodium, 112mg potassium.

Watercress Salad

Yield: 4 servings | **Prep time:** 10 minutes | **Cook time:** 4 minutes

- 2 cups asparagus, chopped
- 16 ounces shrimp, cooked
- 4 cups watercress, torn
- 1 tablespoon apple cider vinegar
- ¼ cup olive oil

1. In the mixing bowl mix up asparagus, shrimps, watercress, and olive oil.
2. T

per serving: 264 calories, 28.3g protein, 4.5g carbohydrates, 14.8g fat, 1.8g fiber, 239mg cholesterol, 300mg sodium, 393mg potassium.

Seafood Arugula Salad

Yield: 4 servings | **Prep time:** 5 minutes | **Cook time:** 10 minutes

- 1 tablespoon olive oil
- 2 cups shrimps, cooked
- 1 cup arugula
- 1 tablespoon cilantro, chopped

1. Put all ingredients in the salad bowl and shake well.

per serving: 61 calories, 6.6g protein, 0.2g carbohydrates, 3.7g fat, 0.1g fiber, 123mg cholesterol, 216mg sodium, 20mg potassium.

Smoked Salad

Yield: 6 servings | **Prep time:** 10 minutes | **Cook time:** 0 minutes

- 1 mango, chopped
- 4 cups lettuce, chopped
- 8 oz smoked turkey, chopped
- 2 tablespoons low-fat yogurt
- 1 teaspoon smoked paprika

1. Mix up all ingredients in the bowls and transfer them in the serving plates.

per serving: 88 calories, 7.1g protein, 11.2g carbohydrates, 1.9g fat, 1.3g fiber, 25mg cholesterol, 350mg sodium, 262mg potassium.

Avocado Salad

Yield: 4 servings | **Prep time:** 5 minutes | **Cook time:** 0 minutes

- ½ teaspoon ground black pepper
- 1 avocado, peeled, pitted and sliced
- 4 cups lettuce, chopped
- 1 cup black olives, pitted and halved
- 1 cup tomatoes, chopped
- 1 tablespoon olive oil

1. Put all ingredients in the salad bowl and mix up well.

per serving: 197 calories, 1.9g protein, 10g carbohydrates, 17.1g fat, 5.4g fiber, 0mg cholesterol, 301mg sodium, 434mg potassium.

Berry Salad with Shrimps

Yield: 4 servings | **Prep time:** 7 minutes | **Cook time:** 0 minutes

- 1 cup corn kernels, cooked
- 1 endive, shredded
- 1 pound shrimp, cooked
- 1 tablespoon lime juice
- 2 cups raspberries, halved
- 2 tablespoons olive oil
- 1 tablespoon parsley, chopped

1. Put all ingredients from the list above in the salad bowl and shake well.

per serving: 283 calories, 29.5g protein, 21.2g carbohydrates, 10.1g fat, 9.1g fiber, 239mg cholesterol, 313mg sodium, 803mg potassium.

Sliced Mushrooms Salad

Yield: 4 servings | **Prep time:** 10 minutes | **Cook time:** 20 minutes

- 1 cup mushrooms, sliced
- 1 tablespoon margarine
- 1 cup lettuce, chopped
- 1 teaspoon lemon juice
- 1 tablespoon fresh dill, chopped
- 1 teaspoon cumin seeds

1. Melt the margarine in the skillet.
2. Add mushrooms and lemon juice. Saute the vegetables for 20 minutes over the medium heat.

3. Then transfer the cooked mushrooms in the salad bowl, add lettuce, dill, and cumin seeds.
4. Stir the salad well.

per serving: 35 calories, 0.9g protein, 1.7g carbohydrates, 3.1g fat, 0.5g fiber, 0mg cholesterol, 38mg sodium, 113mg potassium.

Tender Green Beans Salad

Yield: 8 servings | **Prep time:** 5 minutes | **Cook time:** 0 minutes

- *2 cups green beans, trimmed, chopped, cooked*
- *2 tablespoons olive oil*
- *2 pounds shrimp, cooked, peeled*
- *1 cup tomato, chopped*
- *¼ cup apple cider vinegar*

1. Mix up all ingredients together.
2. Then transfer the salad in the salad bowl.

per serving: 179 calories, 26.5g protein, 4.6g carbohydrates, 5.5g fat, 1.2g fiber, 239mg cholesterol, 280mg sodium, 308mg potassium.

Spinach and Chicken Salad

Yield: 4 servings | **Prep time:** 7 minutes | **Cook time:** 0 minutes

- *1 tablespoon olive oil*
- *A pinch of black pepper*
- *1-pound chicken breast, cooked, skinless, boneless, shredded*
- *1 pound cherry tomatoes, halved*
- *1 red onion, sliced*
- *3 cups spinach, chopped*
- *1 tablespoon lemon juice*
- *1 tablespoon nuts, chopped*

1. Put all ingredients in the salad bowl and gently stir with the help of a spatula.

per serving: 209 calories, 26.4g protein, 8.4g carbohydrates, 7.8g fat, 2.7g fiber, 73mg cholesterol, 97mg sodium, 872mg potassium.

Cilantro Salad

Yield: 4 servings | **Prep time:** 10 minutes | **Cook time:** 8 minutes

- *1 tablespoon avocado oil*
- *1 pound shrimp, peeled and deveined*
- *2 cups lettuce, chopped*
- *1 tablespoon balsamic vinegar*
- *1 tablespoon lemon juice*
- *1 cup fresh cilantro, chopped*

1. Heat up a pan with the oil over medium heat, add the shrimps and cook them for 4 minutes per side or until they are light brown.
2. Transfer the shrimps in the salad bowl and add all remaining ingredients from the list above. Shake the salad.

per serving: 146 calories, 26.1g protein, 3g carbohydrates, 2.5g fat, 0.5g fiber, 239mg cholesterol, 281mg sodium, 270mg potassium.

Iceberg Salad

Yield: 4 servings | **Prep time:** 10 minutes | **Cook time:** 0 minutes

- *1 cup iceberg lettuce, chopped*
- *2 oz scallions, chopped*
- *1 cup carrot, shredded*
- *1 cup radish, sliced*
- *2 tablespoons red vinegar*
- *¼ cup olive oil*

1. Make the dressing: mix up olive oil and red vinegar.
2. Then mix up all remaining ingredients in the salad bowl.
3. Sprinkle the salad with dressing.

per serving: 130 calories, 0.8g protein, 5.1g carbohydrates, 12.7g fat, 1.6g fiber, 0mg cholesterol, 33mg sodium, 214mg potassium.

Seafood Salad with Grapes

Yield: 4 servings | **Prep time:** 5 minutes | **Cook time:** 0 minutes

- *2 tablespoons low-fat mayonnaise*
- *2 teaspoons chili powder*
- *1-pound shrimp, cooked, peeled*
- *1 cup green grapes, halved*
- *1 oz nuts, chopped*

1. Mix up all ingredients in the mixing bowl and transfer the salad in the serving plates.

per serving: 225 calories, 27.4g protein, 9.9g carbohydrates, 8.3g fat, 1.3g fiber, 241mg cholesterol, 390mg sodium, 304mg potassium.

Fennel Bulb Salad

Yield: 4 servings | **Prep time:** 10 minutes | **Cook time:** 0 minutes

- *2 fennel bulbs, chopped*

- *1 cup fresh parsley, chopped*
- *1 tablespoon olive oil*
- *½ cups walnuts, chopped*
- *1 oz low-fat feta cheese, crumbled*
1. Put all ingredients in the salad bowl.
2. Mix up the mixture.

per serving: 181 calories, 6.9g protein, 11.3g carbohydrates, 13.8g fat, 5.2g fiber, 3mg cholesterol, 156mg sodium, 649mg potassium.

Russet Potato Salad

Yield: 4 servings | **Prep time:** 10 minutes | **Cook time:** 20 minutes

- *2 tomatoes, chopped*
- *2 cups spinach, chopped*
- *2 scallions, chopped*
- *3 russet potatoes*
- *1 tablespoon olive oil*
- *1 tablespoon apple cider vinegar*

1. Bake the potatoes in the preheated to 400F oven for 20 minutes.
2. Meanwhile, mix up all remaining ingredients in the salad bowl.
3. Cool the potatoes, peel them, and cut into cubes.
4. Add in the salad and mix up well.

per serving: 158 calories, 3.8g protein, 28.6g carbohydrates, 3.9g fat, 5.1g fiber, 0mg cholesterol, 26mg sodium, 903mg potassium.

Sweet Persimmon Salad

Yield: 4 servings | **Prep time:** 10 minutes | **Cook time:** 0 minutes

- *1/3 cup pomegranate seeds*
- *2 persimmons, chopped*
- *5 cups baby arugula*
- *4 navel oranges, peeled and cut into segments*
- *3 tablespoons pine nuts*
- *2 tablespoons orange juice*
- *¼ teaspoon ground cinnamon*
- *1 tablespoon liquid honey*

1. Put all ingredients in the big salad bowl and mix it up.

per serving: 180 calories, 3.5g protein, 34.8g carbohydrates, 4.9g fat, 5.2g fiber, 0mg cholesterol, 7mg sodium, 521mg potassium.

Mint Seafood Salad

Yield: 4 servings | **Prep time:** 5 minutes | **Cook time:** 18 minutes

- *1 cup of water*
- *2 tablespoons olive oil*
- *2 cups broccoli florets*
- *1 cup shrimps, peeled*
- *4 cherry tomatoes, halved*
- *½ cup kalamata olives, chopped*
- *1 tablespoon mint, chopped*

1. Bring the water to boil, add broccoli, and cook it for 10 minutes.
2. Then add shrimps and cook the ingredients for 5 minutes more.
3. Drain the water and transfer the broccoli and shrimps in the salad bowl.
4. Add all remaining ingredients and shake the salad.

per serving: 118 calories, 2.6g protein, 9g carbohydrates, 9.2g fat, 3.3g fiber, 0mg cholesterol, 170mg sodium, 444mg potassium.

Green Dill Salad

Yield: 4 servings | **Prep time:** 10 minutes | **Cook time:** 4 minutes

- *½ cup dill, chopped*
- *1 cup asparagus, chopped*
- *1 tablespoon olive oil*
- *1 tablespoon lemon juice*
- *1 tablespoon canola oil*
- *1 teaspoon sesame seeds*
- *1 cup lettuce, chopped*

1. Roast the asparagus with olive oil in the skillet for 4 minutes and transfer it in the salad bowl.
2. Add all remaining ingredients and stir the salad well.

per serving: 90 calories, 2.2g protein, 5.3g carbohydrates, 7.7g fat, 1.7g fiber, 0mg cholesterol, 15mg sodium, 294mg potassium.

Fish and Mushrooms Salad

Yield: 4 servings | **Prep time:** 10 minutes | **Cook time:** 20 minutes

- *2 salmon fillets, chopped*
- *1 tablespoon olive oil*
- *½ teaspoon oregano, dried*
- *8 ounces white mushrooms, sliced*
- *1 tablespoon lemon juice*
- *1 cup black olives, pitted and halved*
- *1 tablespoon parsley, chopped*

- ½ cup of water
1. Put salmon and mushrooms in the baking pan.
2. Add water and oregano. Bake the ingredients for 20 minutes at 365F.
3. Then transfer the cooked ingredients in the salad bowl.
4. Add all remaining ingredients and mix up.

per serving: 211 calories, 20g protein, 2.4g carbohydrates, 13.4g fat, 1.2g fiber, 55mg cholesterol, 339mg sodium, 500mg potassium.

Tropical Salad

Yield: 4 servings | **Prep time:** 10 minutes | **Cook time:** 30 minutes

- 2 cups pineapple, chopped
- 4 potatoes, cubed
- 1 tablespoon olive oil
- 1/3 cup almonds, chopped
- 2 tablespoons low-fat cream cheese

1. Bake potatoes at 390F for 30 minutes or until soft.
2. Then mix up cooked potatoes with pineapple, olive oil, almonds, and cream cheese.

per serving: 281 calories, 6.1g protein, 46.1g carbohydrates, 9.5g fat, 7.3g fiber, 6mg cholesterol, 29mg sodium, 1021mg potassium.

Spring Salad

Yield: 4 servings | **Prep time:** 0 minutes | **Cook time:** 0 minutes

- 3 oz scallions, chopped
- 1 tablespoon chives, chopped
- 3 cups radish, sliced
- 1 tablespoon low-fat yogurt
- ½ teaspoon ground black pepper

1. Put all ingredients in the salad bowl and mix it up.

per serving: 24 calories, 1.3g protein, 5g carbohydrates, 0.2g fat, 2g fiber, 0mg cholesterol, 40mg sodium, 276mg potassium.

Tender Endives Salad

Yield: 4 servings | **Prep time:** 5 minutes | **Cook time:** 0 minutes

- 2 heads endives, chopped
- 1 tablespoon parsley, chopped
- 2 tablespoons lemon juice
- 2 tablespoons olive oil
- 2 cups arugula, chopped

1. Put all ingredients from the list above in the salad bowl and stir well.

per serving: 108 calories, 3.6g protein, 9.2g carbohydrates, 7.7g fat, 8.2g fiber, 0mg cholesterol, 61mg sodium, 857mg potassium.

Bean Sprouts Salad

Yield: 4 servings | **Prep time:** 10 minutes | **Cook time:** 0 minutes

- 2 cups bean sprouts
- ½ cup bell pepper, chopped
- 1 tablespoon olive oil
- ½ cup cilantro, chopped
- 2 pecans, chopped

1. Put all ingredients in the salad bowl and mix it up.

per serving: 111 calories, 4.8g protein, 6g carbohydrates, 9g fat, 1g fiber, 0mg cholesterol, 7mg sodium, 239mg potassium.

Pine Nuts Salad

Yield: 4 servings | **Prep time:** 5 minutes | **Cook time:** 0 minutes

- 5 cups baby arugula
- 2 tablespoons chives, chopped
- 1 tablespoon balsamic vinegar
- 2 tablespoons avocado oil
- 3 tablespoons pine nuts

1. Combine together all ingredients in the salad bowl and cool in the fridge for 3 minutes.

per serving: 60 calories, 1.7g protein, 2.2g carbohydrates, 5.5g fat, 1g fiber, 0mg cholesterol, 7mg sodium, 160mg potassium.

Cucumber and Lettuce Salad

Yield: 4 servings | **Prep time:** 5 minutes | **Cook time:** 0 minutes

- 2 cups romaine lettuce, roughly chopped
- 1 cup corn kernels, cooked
- ½ pound green beans, cooked, roughly chopped
- 1 cup cucumber, chopped
- 1 tablespoon canola oil

1. Mix up all ingredients in the salad bowl and transfer the salad in the serving plates, if desired.

per serving: 89 calories, 2.6g protein, 13.1g carbohydrates, 4.1g fat, 3.3g fiber, 0mg cholesterol, 11mg sodium, 300mg potassium.

Endive-Kale Salad

Yield: 4 servings | **Prep time:** 5 minutes | **Cook time:** 4 minutes
- 1 head endives, chopped
- 2 tablespoons lime juice
- 1 tablespoon sesame oil
- 1 teaspoon sesame seeds
- 1 tablespoon balsamic vinegar
- 2 cups kale, chopped

1. Place all ingredients in the salad bowl and stir the salad well.

per serving: 75 calories, 2.8g protein, 8.5g carbohydrates, 4.1g fat, 4.6g fiber, 0mg cholesterol, 44mg sodium, 579mg potassium.

Garlic Edamame Salad

Yield: 4 servings | **Prep time:** 7 minutes | **Cook time:** 0 minutes
- 2 tablespoons avocado oil
- 2 tablespoons apple cider vinegar
- 1 teaspoon minced garlic
- 2 cups edamame, cooked
- 2 tablespoons scallions, chopped

1. Stir together all ingredients in the salad bowl.
2. Cool aside the salad for 5 minutes.

per serving: 201 calories, 16.8g protein, 15.1g carbohydrates, 9.6g fat, 5.8g fiber, 0mg cholesterol, 20mg sodium, 832mg potassium.

Orange Mango Salad

Yield: 4 servings | **Prep time:** 7 minutes | **Cook time:** 0 minutes
- 1 cup mango, peeled and cubed
- 2 cups oranges, chopped
- 1 tablespoon low-fat yogurt
- 2 tablespoons walnuts, chopped
- 1 teaspoon vanilla extract

1. Put all ingredients in the bowl and mix up well.
2. Then transfer the salad in the serving bowls.

per serving: 97 calories, 2.4g protein, 17.6g carbohydrates, 2.6g fat, 3.1g fiber, 0g cholesterol, 3mg sodium, 263mg potassium.

Garden Salad

Yield: 4 servings | **Prep time:** 5 minutes | **Cook time:** 0 minutes
- 2 shallots, chopped
- 2 carrots, grated
- 1 big red cabbage head, shredded
- 1 tablespoon olive oil
- 1 tablespoon red vinegar
- A pinch of black pepper
- 1 tablespoon lime juice

1. Mix up all salad ingredients in the salad bowl and cool aside for 2-3 minutes in the fridge.

per serving: 97 calories, 2.4g protein, 17.6g carbohydrates, 2.6g fat, 3.1g fiber, 0mg cholesterol, 3mg sodium, 263mg potassium.

Dinner Salad

Yield: 4 servings | **Prep time:** 7 minutes | **Cook time:** 0 minutes
- 10 oz tuna, canned, shredded
- ¼ cup green onions, chopped
- 2 cups fresh spinach, chopped
- 1 tablespoon low-fat parmesan, grated
- 1 tablespoon low-fat yogurt
- ½ teaspoon ground black pepper

1. Make a dressing: mix up yogurt with ground black pepper and green onions.
2. Then mix up all remaining ingredients in the salad bowl and top with dressing.

per serving: 144 calories, 19.8g protein, 1.5g carbohydrates, 6.1g fat, 0.6g fiber, 23mg cholesterol, 70mg sodium, 351mg potassium.

Tomato and Beef Salad

Yield: 4 servings | **Prep time:** 10 minutes | **Cook time:** 20 minutes
- 1 cup tomatoes, chopped
- 2 avocados, pitted and chopped
- 2 cups lean ground beef
- 1 teaspoon chili flakes
- 1 onion, diced
- 1 tablespoon olive oil
- 1 teaspoon dried oregano

1. Heat up the olive oil in the skillet.
2. Add onion and cook it for 5 minutes.
3. Then add lean ground beef and oregano. Cook the meat for 15 minutes.
4. Then cool it little and mix up with tomatoes, avocado, and chili flakes.
5. Shake the salad gently.

per serving: 385 calories,15.7g protein, 13.2g carbohydrates, 31.4g fat, 8g fiber, 45mg cholesterol, 57mg sodium, 808mg potassium.

Avocado Sweet Salad

Yield: 4 servings | **Prep time:** 10 minutes | **Cook time:** 0 minutes

- 2 tablespoons of liquid honey
- 2 tablespoon apple cider vinegar
- 1 avocado, peeled, pitted and chopped
- 4 cups baby spinach
- 1 cup tangerines, chopped
- 2 teaspoons sesame seeds, toasted

1. Mix up all ingredients except sesame seeds in the salad bowl and stir well.
2. Top the salad with sesame seeds.

per serving: 175 calories,2.5g protein, 20.4g carbohydrates, 10.7g fat, 4.7g fiber, 0mg cholesterol, 31mg sodium, 512mg potassium.

Dinner Shrimp Salad

Yield: 4 servings | **Prep time:** 10 minutes | **Cook time:** 10 minutes

- 2 cups asparagus, chopped
- 1 cup corn kernels, cooked
- 1 cup shrimps, peeled
- 1 tablespoon olive oil
- 1 teaspoon sesame oil
- 1 tablespoon lemon juice
- 1 teaspoon Italian seasonings

1. Mix up shrimps, asparagus, Italian seasonings, and olive oil in the tray and bake at 375F for 10 minutes.
2. Then transfer the cooked ingredients in the salad bowl.
3. Add all remaining ingredients and mix up well.

per serving: 206 calories,9.5g protein, 22.8g carbohydrates, 9.5g fat, 3.2g fiber, 1mg cholesterol, 8mg sodium, 245mg potassium.

Vegan Salad

Yield: 4 servings | **Prep time:** 10 minutes | **Cook time:** 0 minutes

- 1 pound firm tofu, drained and cubed
- 1 tablespoon olive oil
- 1 cup bell pepper, chopped
- 1 cup cucumbers, chopped
- ½ cup sorrel leaves, torn

1. Put all ingredients in the serving bowl and stir well.

per serving: 123 calories,9.8g protein, 5.1g carbohydrates, 8.3g fat, 1.6g fiber, 0mg cholesterol, 15mg sodium, 262mg potassium.

Green Cabbage Salad

Yield: 6 servings | **Prep time:** 60 minutes | **Cook time:** 0 minutes

- 4 cups green cabbage, shredded
- 2 carrots, shredded
- 1 cup radish, chopped
- 1 red onion, diced
- 2 tablespoons olive oil
- ¼ cup apple cider vinegar
- 1 teaspoon ground black pepper

1. Put all ingredients in the glass jar and shake well.
2. Close the lid and leave the salad in the cold place for 50 minutes.

per serving: 73 calories,1.1g protein, 7.4g carbohydrates, 4.8g fat, 2.5g fiber, 0mg cholesterol, 31mg sodium, 228mg potassium.

Grilled Tofu Salad

Yield: 3 servings | **Prep time:** 15 minutes | **Cook time:** 4 minutes

- 8 oz tofu, cubed
- 1 teaspoon curry paste
- 3 tablespoons low-fat milk
- 1 teaspoon sesame oil
- 1 cup lettuce, chopped
- 1 cup cherry tomatoes, halved
- 1 tablespoon lemon juice

1. Mix up curry paste, tofu, and milk in the bowl and leave for 10 minutes to marinate.
2. Then place the tofu in the preheated to 400F grill and cook it for 2 minutes per side.
3. Meanwhile, mix up the remaining ingredients from the list above.
4. Top the salad with grilled tofu and shake gently.

per serving: 98 calories,7.4g protein, 5.5g carbohydrates, 6g fat, 1.5g fiber, 1mg cholesterol, 21mg sodium, 309mg potassium.

Balsamic Vinegar Salad

Yield: 3 servings | **Prep time:** 10 minutes | **Cook time:** 0 minutes

- 2 cups lettuce, chopped
- 2 cups cucumbers, chopped

- ¼ cup balsamic vinegar
- 1 teaspoon mustard
- 1 teaspoon olive oil

1. Make the dressing: mix mustard, olive oil, and balsamic vinegar.
2. Then mix up lettuce and cucumbers in the salad bowl.
3. Top the salad with dressing and shake well.

per serving: 38 calories, 0.9g protein, 4.2g carbohydrates, 2g fat, 0.7g fiber, 0mg cholesterol, 4mg sodium, 176mg potassium.

Mint Cauliflower Salad

Yield: 4 servings | **Prep time:** 10 minutes | **Cook time:** 10 minutes

- 1 cup of water
- 2 cups cauliflower, chopped
- 1 teaspoon dried mint
- 2 tablespoons olive oil
- 2 cups fresh cilantro, chopped
- 1 red onion, diced
- 2 tablespoons lemon juice
- 1 teaspoon white pepper

1. Boil the cauliflower in water for 10 minutes.
2. Then drain the water and cool the cauliflower.
3. Transfer it in the salad bowl.
4. Add all remaining ingredients and shake well.

per serving: 89 calories, 1.6g protein, 6.1g carbohydrates, 7.2g fat, 2.3g fiber, 0mg cholesterol, 23mg sodium, 252mg potassium.

Butternut Squash Salad

Yield: 6 servings | **Prep time:** 10 minutes | **Cook time:** 30 minutes

- 1 cup of orange juice
- 1 teaspoon liquid honey
- ½ teaspoon ground cinnamon
- ½ tablespoons mustard
- 2-pound butternut squash, peeled, chopped
- 1 cup banana, chopped
- 1 tablespoon lemon juice

1. Mix up butternut squash with ground cinnamon and liquid honey and bake for 30 minutes at 365F.
2. Then transfer the cooked vegetable in the salad bowl.
3. Add mustard, banana, and lemon juice.
4. Shake the salad well.

per serving: 127 calories, 2.8g protein, 29.8g carbohydrates, 1.1g fat, 4.3g fiber, 0mg cholesterol, 7mg sodium, 728mg potassium.

Poultry

Chicken Skillet

Yield: 6 servings | **Prep time:** 10 minutes | **Cook time:** 26 minutes

- 4 chicken fillets
- 1 teaspoon ground black pepper
- ½ teaspoon ground paprika
- 1 tablespoon olive oil
- 3 oz low-fat sour cream
- 1 cup asparagus, chopped
- ¼ cup of water

1. Slice the chicken fillet and sprinkle it with ground black pepper and paprika.
2. Put the sliced chicken in the skillet, add olive oil, and cook it for 3 minutes from each side.
3. Then add low-fat sour cream and asparagus.
4. Add water and close the lid.
5. Saute the meal for 20 minutes.

per serving: 241 calories, 29.2g protein, 1.8g carbohydrates, 12.6g fat, 0.6g fiber, 93mg cholesterol, 92mg sodium, 311mg potassium.

Turkey Stir-Fry

Yield: 5 servings | **Prep time:** 10 minutes | **Cook time:** 25 minutes

- 12 oz turkey fillet, sliced
- 1 carrot, julienned
- 1 onion, sliced
- 1 teaspoon potato starch
- ½ cup low-sodium chicken broth
- 1 teaspoon chili powder
- 1 tablespoon avocado oil

1. Pour avocado oil in the saucepan and add turkey fillet.
2. Roast the poultry for 2 minutes from each side.
3. Then add carrot, onion, and chili powder. Stir the ingredients and cook them for 10 minutes.
4. Meanwhile, mix up chicken broth and potato starch.
5. Pour the liquid over the turkey mixture and stir well.

6. Cook the meal for 10 minutes more.
per serving: 89 calories, 14.8g protein, 4.8g carbohydrates, 0.8g fat, 1.1g fiber, 35mg cholesterol, 176mg sodium, 90mg potassium.

Chicken and Low-fat Goat Cheese Bowl

Yield: 4 servings | **Prep time:** 10 minutes | **Cook time:** 20 minutes
- 1-pound chicken breast, skinless, boneless, chopped
- 2 tomatoes, chopped
- 3 oz low-fat goat cheese, crumbled
- ½ teaspoon ground black pepper
- ¼ teaspoon garlic powder
- 1 tablespoon olive oil
- 1 tablespoon lemon juice

1. Mix up the chicken with olive oil, lemon juice, garlic powder, and ground black pepper.
2. Then transfer the chicken in the baking tray, flatten it well and bake at 400F for 20 minutes.
3. After this, put the cooked chicken in the serving bowls and top with tomatoes and low-fat goat cheese.

per serving: 269 calories, 31.2g protein, 3.2g carbohydrates, 14.1g fat, 0.9g fiber, 95mg cholesterol, 135mg sodium, 586mg potassium.

Chicken Chop Suey

Yield: 4 servings | **Prep time:** 10 minutes | **Cook time:** 35 minutes
- ¼ cup reduced-sodium soy sauce
- 1-pound chicken fillet, chopped
- ½ cup mushrooms, chopped
- ½ onion, chopped
- ½ teaspoon chili flakes
- 2 tablespoons avocado oil
- 1 cup bean sprouts, canned

1. Heat up avocado oil in the deep skillet.
2. Add mushrooms and roast them for 3 minutes.
3. Then add chopped onion, stir the vegetables and cook them for 7 minutes. Stir them from time to time to avoid burning.
4. Transfer the cooked vegetables in the serving bowls.
5. Then add chicken in the skillet and sprinkle it with chili flakes. Cook it for 15 minutes. Stir it occasionally.
6. Then add bean sprouts and cook the meal for 10 minutes more.
7. Transfer the chicken mixture over the mushroom-onion mixture.

per serving: 169 calories, 24.1g protein, 3.5g carbohydrates, 6.4g fat, 0.6g fiber, 67mg cholesterol, 422mg sodium, 307mg potassium.

Chicken Packets

Yield: 3 servings | **Prep time:** 15 minutes | **Cook time:** 35 minutes
- 12 oz chicken fillet
- 2 sweet peppers, sliced
- 1 red onion, sliced
- 1 teaspoon Italian seasonings
- 2 tablespoons olive oil
- 1 tomato, sliced
- 3 tablespoons apple cider vinegar

1. Cut the chicken fillet on 3 servings.
2. Then place them in the 3 baking packets.
3. Add sliced sweet pepper, onion, Italian seasonings, olive oil, tomato, and apple cider vinegar. Secure the packets and shake well.
4. Preheat the oven to 385F.
5. Put the chicken packets in the tray and bake them for 35 minutes.

per serving: 347 calories, 34.2g protein, 10.2g carbohydrates, 18.5g fat, 2.1g fiber, 102mg cholesterol, 103mg sodium, 539+mg potassium.

Herbed Chicken Breast

Yield: 4 servings | **Prep time:** 10 minutes | **Cook time:** 45 minutes
- 1-pound chicken breast
- 1 teaspoon dried sage
- 1 teaspoon dried basil
- 1 teaspoon ground paprika
- 1 teaspoon dried oregano
- ¼ teaspoon cumin seeds
- 2 tablespoons margarine, melted

1. In the shallow bowl mix up sage, basil, paprika, oregano, and cumin seeds.
2. Rub the chicken with the spice mixture and then generously brush with the melted margarine.

3. Wrap the chicken breast in the foil and bake in the preheated to 375F oven for 45 minutes.
per serving: 184 calories, 24.3g protein, 0.8g carbohydrates, 8.7g fat, 0.4g fiber, 73mg cholesterol, 125mg sodium, 446mg potassium.

Chicken and Vegetables Wraps

Yield: 3 servings | **Prep time:** 10 minutes | **Cook time:** 8 minutes
- 3 lettuce leaves
- 9 oz chicken fillet
- 1 teaspoon rotisserie chicken seasonings
- 3 celery stalks
- 1 carrot, cut into sticks
- 3 teaspoons low-fat yogurt
- 1 tablespoon olive oil

1. Slice the chicken and put it in the skillet.
2. Add olive oil and roast it for 4 minutes from each side or until the chicken slices are light brown.
3. Then cool the chicken gently and place it on the lettuce leaves.
4. Add celery stalks and carrot. Sprinkle the ingredients with yogurt and wrap.

per serving: 217 calories, 25.2g protein, 3g carbohydrates, 11.1g fat, 0.8g fiber, 76mg cholesterol, 122mg sodium, 335mg potassium.

Sesame Shredded Chicken

Yield: 2 servings | **Prep time:** 10 minutes | **Cook time:** 20 minutes
- 10 oz chicken breast, skinless, boneless
- 1 cup of water
- 1 teaspoon sesame seeds
- 1 teaspoon sesame oil
- 1 tomato, chopped
- ½ teaspoon cayenne pepper

1. Put the chicken breast in water and boil it for 15 minutes.
2. Then drain water and shred the chicken.
3. Transfer the shredded chicken in the skillet.
4. Add sesame oil, cayenne pepper, and tomato.
5. Cook the shredded chicken for 5 minutes.
6. Sprinkle the cooked meal with sesame seeds.

per serving: 197 calories, 30.6g protein, 1.8g carbohydrates, 6.7g fat, 0.7g fiber, 91mg cholesterol, 78mg sodium, 615mg potassium.

Chicken Piccata

Yield: 3 servings | **Prep time:** 10 minutes | **Cook time:** 12 minutes
- 9 oz chicken fillet
- 1 tablespoon whole-grain wheat flour
- 1 teaspoon ground black pepper
- 3 tablespoons lemon juice
- 1/3 cup low-sodium chicken stock
- 1 teaspoon margarine
- 1 tablespoon capers

1. Chop the chicken fillet and sprinkle with flour.
2. Then melt the margarine in the skillet, add chicken and roast it for 2 minutes from each side.
3. After this, add ground black pepper, lemon juice, chicken stock, and capers.
4. Stir the chicken well and close the lid.
5. Cook the chicken piccata for 5-7 minutes more.

per serving: 188 calories, 25.3g protein, 2.7g carbohydrates, 7.8g fat, 0.7g fiber, 76mg cholesterol, 192mg sodium, 246mg potassium.

Lean Chicken Thighs

Yield: 4 servings | **Prep time:** 10 minutes | **Cook time:** 25 minutes
- ½ teaspoon ground black pepper
- ½ teaspoon ground paprika
- ½ teaspoon garlic powder
- 1 tablespoon sesame oil
- 4 chicken thighs, boneless, skinless

1. Rub the chicken thighs with ground black pepper, paprika, and garlic powder.
2. The heat up the skillet and pour oil inside.
3. Add chicken thighs and cook them for 10 minutes. Flip the chicken on another side and cook for 10 minutes more.

per serving: 310 calories, 42.4g protein, 0.6g carbohydrates, 14.3g fat, 0.2g fiber, 130mg cholesterol, 126mg sodium, 368mg potassium.

Blackened Chicken

Yield: 2 servings | **Prep time:** 10 minutes | **Cook time:** 25 minutes
- 8 oz chicken fillet
- ½ teaspoon ground coriander
- ½ teaspoon ground cumin
- 1 teaspoon ground paprika
- 1 teaspoon dried oregano
- ½ teaspoon ground black pepper
- 1 tablespoon olive oil
- 1 teaspoon water

1. Cut the chicken fillet on 2 servings and sprinkle with water.
2. In the mixing bowl, mix up all spices from the list above.
3. Heat up the olive oil in the skillet.
4. Then rub the chicken fillets with the spice mix and put in the hot oil.
5. Roast chicken for 5 minutes from each side.
6. Then transfer it in the baking tray and cook for 15 minutes more at 385F.

per serving: 284calories,33.2g protein, 1.6g carbohydrates, 15.8g fat, 0.9g fiber, 101mg cholesterol, 99mg sodium, 329mg potassium.

Grilled Chicken Fillets

Yield: 6 servings | **Prep time:** 15 minutes | **Cook time:** 15minutes
- 18 oz chicken fillet
- 1 teaspoon cumin seeds
- 2 tablespoons olive oil
- 1/2 teaspoon dried sage
- 1 teaspoon dried basil
- ½ lemon

1. Squeeze the juice from the lemon in the bowl.
2. Add cumin seeds, olive oil, sage, and basil.
3. Then cut the chicken fillet on 6 servings and place in the lemon mixture.
4. Marinate the chicken or 10-15 minutes.
5. Meanwhile, preheat the grill to 400F.
6. Put the marinated chicken in the grill and cook for 7 minutes from each side.
7. Slice the chicken and transfer in the serving plates.

per serving: 205 calories,27.4g protein, 0.6g carbohydrates, 11.1g fat, 0.2g fiber, 76mg cholesterol, 74mg sodium, 221mg potassium.

Oregano Turkey Tenders

Yield: 4 servings | **Prep time:** 10 minutes | **Cook time:** 10 minutes
- 2 turkey breast fillets, skinless, boneless
- 1 tablespoon dried oregano
- 1 tablespoon olive oil

1. Cut the chicken fillets into the tenders and sprinkle with dried oregano and olive oil.
2. Then put the turkey tenders in the skillet in one layer and cook them for 5 minutes from each side or until the tenders are golden brown.

per serving: 101 calories,13.5g protein, 1.2g carbohydrates, 4.8g fat, 0.2g fiber, 30mg cholesterol, 240mg sodium, 6mg potassium.

Turkey Chili

Yield: 6 servings | **Prep time:** 10 minutes | **Cook time:** 35 minutes
- 2 cups ground turkey
- 1 cup red kidney beans, canned
- 1 cup tomatoes, chopped
- 1 teaspoon chili powder
- ½ teaspoon ground cayenne pepper
- 3 cups of water
- 1 tablespoon margarine
- 1 onion, diced

1. Toss margarine in the saucepan and melt it.
2. Add onion and cook it for 3 minutes.
3. Then stir it and add ground turkey.
4. Sprinkle the turkey with chili powder and ground cayenne pepper. Stir well and cook for 5 minutes.
5. Add red kidney beans, tomatoes, and water.
6. Close the lid and cook chili for 30 minutes over the medium heat.

per serving: 349 calories,37.6g protein, 22g carbohydrates, 14.5g fat, 5.6g fiber, 112mg cholesterol, 154mg sodium, 825mg potassium.

Turkey Bake

Yield: 4 servings | **Prep time:** 15 minutes | **Cook time:** 45 minutes
- 1 cup broccoli, chopped
- ¼ cup low-fat cheese, shredded
- 1 cup ground turkey
- 1 teaspoon chili flakes
- 1 cup low-fat sour cream
- 1 teaspoon olive oil

- 1 jalapeno pepper, chopped
1. Brush the casserole mold with olive oil. Preheat the oven to 390F.
2. Then mix up ground turkey and chili flakes and transfer the mixture in the prepared casserole mold. Flatten the mixture well.
3. After this, top it with broccoli, jalapeno pepper, and low-fat sour cream.
4. Sprinkle the mixture with the shredded cheese and top with foil.
5. Bake the meal for 45 minutes.

per serving: 211 calories, 24.3g protein, 7.8g carbohydrates, 9.2g fat, 0.7g fiber, 64mg cholesterol, 144mg sodium, 335mg potassium.

Turkey Meatloaf

Yield: 6 servings | **Prep time:** 15 minutes | **Cook time:** 35 minutes
- 1-pound ground turkey
- 2 oz walnuts, chopped
- 1 teaspoon Italian seasonings
- 1 tablespoon potato starch
- 1 tablespoon semolina
- ¼ cup corn kernels
- 1 teaspoon olive oil

1. In the mixing bowl mix up ground turkey, walnuts, Italian seasonings, potato starch, semolina, and corn kernels.
2. Then brush the meatloaf mold with olive oil and put the turkey mixture inside.
3. Flatten it well and cover with the foil.
4. Transfer the meatloaf in the preheated to 380F oven and cook it 35 minutes.

per serving: 233 calories, 23.4g protein, 5.2g carbohydrates, 15g fat, 0.9g fiber, 78mg cholesterol, 82mg sodium, 275mg potassium.

Turkey Burgers

Yield: 3 servings | **Prep time:** 10 minutes | **Cook time:** 10 minutes
- 9 oz ground turkey
- ¼ cup fresh parsley, chopped
- 1 teaspoon minced garlic
- ½ teaspoon chili pepper
- 1 tablespoon semolina
- 1 tablespoon coconut oil

1. Mix up ground turkey, parsley, garlic, chili pepper, and semolina.
2. Heat up coconut oil in the skillet.
3. After this, make the burgers and put them in the hot coconut oil.
4. Cook the burgers for 4 minutes per side.

per serving: 221 calories, 23.9g protein, 3.3g carbohydrates, 14g fat, 0.4g fiber, 87mg cholesterol, 94mg sodium, 270mg potassium.

Curry Chicken Wings

Yield: 4 servings | **Prep time:** 10 minutes | **Cook time:** 25 minutes
- 1-pound chicken wings, skinless, boneless
- 1 teaspoon curry paste
- ½ cup skim milk
- 1 tablespoon coconut oil

1. Mix up skim milk and curry paste until smooth.
2. Then toss the coconut oil in the saucepan and melt it.
3. Add the chicken wings and cook them for 2 minutes per side.
4. After this, add curry paste mixture and stir the chicken.
5. Close the lid and cook the meal for 20 minutes on medium heat.

per serving: 264 calories, 33.9g protein, 1.9g carbohydrates, 12.5g fat, 0g fiber, 102mg cholesterol, 114mg sodium, 323mg potassium.

Basil Stuffed Chicken Breast

Yield: 4 servings | **Prep time:** 15 minutes | **Cook time:** 45 minutes
- 1 tomato, sliced
- 1 oz basil leaves
- 1 teaspoon ground black pepper
- 1 tablespoon sesame oil
- 1 teaspoon minced garlic
- 1-pound chicken breast, skinless, boneless

1. Make the lengthwise cut in the chicken breast.
2. Then rub the chicken breast with minced garlic, ground black pepper, and fill with basil leaves and tomato slices.
3. Secure the cut with toothpicks.
4. Then brush the chicken breast with sesame oil and wrap in the foil.
5. Bake the chicken for 45 minutes at 385F.

per serving: 166 calories, 24.5g protein, 1.4g carbohydrates, 6.3g fat, 0.5g fiber, 73mg cholesterol, 59mg sodium, 487mg potassium.

Tomato Chicken Stew

Yield: 4 servings | **Prep time:** 10 minutes | **Cook time:** 25 minutes
- 10 oz chicken fillet, chopped
- 2 sweet peppers, chopped
- 1 cup tomatoes, chopped
- 1 chili pepper, chopped
- ¼ cup of water
- 1 teaspoon olive oil

1. Heat up olive oil in the skillet.
2. Add sweet pepper and chili pepper. Roast the vegetables for 3 minutes.
3. After this, add chicken and cook the ingredients for 10 minutes.
4. Add tomatoes and water.
5. Stir the stew well and cook it for 10 minutes more.

per serving: 172 calories, 21.5g protein, 6.3g carbohydrates, 6.7g fat, 1.4g fiber, 63mg cholesterol, 65mg sodium, 393mg potassium.

Turkey Mix

Yield: 4 servings | **Prep time:** 5 minutes | **Cook time:** 25 minutes
- 2 tablespoons canola oil
- 1-pound turkey fillet, sliced
- ½ teaspoon ground black pepper
- 3 garlic cloves, minced
- 1 cup artichoke, canned, chopped
- 1 cup low-fat milk

1. Heat up a pan with the oil over medium-high heat, add sliced turkey, garlic and the black pepper, cook the ingredients for 5 minutes.
2. Add the rest of the ingredients, toss and cook over medium heat for 15 minutes.
3. Stir well and cook for 5 minutes more.

per serving: 232 calories, 30.8g protein, 7.2g carbohydrates, 8.3g fat, 1.9 fiber, 72mg cholesterol, 357mg sodium, 222mg potassium.

Onion Chicken

Yield: 4 servings | **Prep time:** 10 minutes | **Cook time:** 45 minutes
- 3 tablespoons olive oil
- 1 cup onion, chopped
- 1-pound chicken breast, skinless, boneless
- ½ teaspoon oregano, dried
- 1 cup of water
- 1 tablespoon parsley, chopped

1. Heat up a pan with 2 tablespoons of olive oil over medium-low heat, add the onion, and cook it for 10 minutes.
2. Add all remaining ingredients except water and cook the meal for 15 minutes more.
3. Then add water, stir well and cook the chicken for 20 minutes.

per serving: 232 calories, 24.4g protein, 2.9g carbohydrates, 13.4g fat, 0.7g fiber, 73mg cholesterol, 61mg sodium, 471mg potassium.

Spiced Turkey Fillet

Yield: 4 servings | **Prep time:** 10 minutes | **Cook time:** 30 minutes
- 2 tablespoons canola oil
- 1 red onion, chopped
- 2 tablespoons oregano
- 1-pound turkey fillet, chopped
- ½ cup of water

6. Heat up canola oil in the saucepan.
7. Add turkey, oregano, and onion and cook the ingredients for 5 minutes.
8. Then add water and close the lid.
9. Simmer the meal for 25 minutes over medium heat.

per serving: 187 calories, 24.1g protein, 4g carbohydrates, 7.8g fat, 1.6g fiber, 59mg cholesterol, 259mg sodium, 78mg potassium.

Balsamic Vinegar Chicken

Yield: 4 servings | **Prep time:** 10 minutes | **Cook time:** 35 minutes
- 1 tablespoon olive oil
- 1-pound chicken breast, skinless, boneless
- 1/3 cup balsamic vinegar
- 2 teaspoons thyme, chopped
- 1 teaspoon rosemary, chopped
- 1 teaspoon lemon zest, grated

1. Heat up a pan with the oil over medium-high heat, add chicken and cook for 5 minutes and transfer to a plate.
2. Heat up the same pan over medium heat, add all remaining ingredients and bring the mixture to boil.
3. Return chicken to the pan and cook the meal for 10 minutes.
4. Then bake the meal at 325F for 25 minutes.

per serving: 166 calories, 24.1g protein, 0.8g carbohydrates, 6.4g fat, 0.4g fiber, 73mg cholesterol, 59mg sodium, 443mg potassium.

Citrus Chicken

Yield: 4 servings | **Prep time:** 10 minutes | **Cook time:** 35 minutes

- 1 tablespoon avocado oil
- 1 pound chicken breast, skinless, boneless, roughly chopped
- 1 orange, chopped
- ½ cup of orange juice
- 1 tablespoon orange zest, grated
- 1 teaspoon ground black pepper
- ½ teaspoon ground turmeric

1. Heat up a pan with the oil over medium-high heat, add chicken and cook for 5 minutes.
2. Add the rest of the ingredients, toss, and bake in the oven at 340F for 30 minutes.

per serving: 173 calories, 24.8g protein, 9.7g carbohydrates, 3.5g fat, 1.7g fiber, 73mg cholesterol, 59mg sodium, 593mg potassium.

Glazed Chicken

Yield: 8 servings | **Prep time:** 10 minutes | **Cook time:** 30 minutes

- 8 chicken thighs, boneless and skinless
- ½ cup balsamic vinegar
- 3 tablespoon garlic, minced
- 1 teaspoon ground black pepper
- 3 tablespoons hot chili sauce

1. Put the oil in a baking dish, add chicken, and remaining ingredients.
2. Toss well and bake at 425F for 30 minutes.

per serving: 286 calories, 42.5g protein, 1.4g carbohydrates, 10.9g fat, 0.2g fiber, 130mg cholesterol, 270mg sodium, 389mg potassium.

Turkey Mushrooms

Yield: 4 servings | **Prep time:** 10 minutes | **Cook time:** 40 minutes

- 1-pound turkey fillet, sliced
- ½ pound white mushrooms, halved
- 1 teaspoon minced garlic
- 2 tablespoons olive oil
- ½ onion, diced
- 1/3 cup water
- 1 tablespoon rosemary, chopped

1. Heat up a pan with the oil over medium heat, add the onions, and the garlic and sauté for 5 minutes.
2. Add the remaining ingredients and stir well.
3. Then transfer the meal in the preheated to 390F for 30 minutes.

per serving: 188 calories, 25.6g protein, 3.9g carbohydrates, 7.8g fat, 1.2g fiber, 59mg cholesterol, 262mg sodium, 211mg potassium.

Spring Chicken Mix

Yield: 4 servings | **Prep time:** 10 minutes | **Cook time:** 25 minutes

- 1 tablespoon sesame oil
- 1-pound chicken breast, skinless, boneless, chopped
- ½ teaspoon white pepper
- 1 shallot, chopped
- 2 garlic cloves, minced
- 1 cup radish, chopped
- 1 cup spinach, chopped
- 2 cups of water

1. Heat up olive oil in the saucepan.
2. Add chicken and roast it for 10 minutes.
3. Then add all remaining ingredients, close the lid, and cook the meal for 15 minutes more.

per serving: 169 calories, 24.6g protein, 2g carbohydrates, 6.3g fat, 0.7g fiber, 73mg cholesterol, 79mg sodium, 540mg potassium.

Peach Turkey

Yield: 4 servings | **Prep time:** 10 minutes | **Cook time:** 25 minutes

- 1 tablespoon olive oil
- 1 1-pound turkey fillet, chopped
- 1 teaspoon chili powder
- 1 cup peaches, chopped
- 1 teaspoon ground paprika
- 1 cup of water

1. Roast the turkey with olive oil in the saucepan for 5 minutes.
2. Then add all remaining ingredients and stir well.
3. Cook the meal for 20 minutes over the medium heat.

per serving: 155 calories, 24.1g protein, 4.2g carbohydrates, 4.3g fat, 1g fiber, 59mg cholesterol, 264mg sodium, 96mg potassium.

Chicken with Vegetables

Yield: 4 servings | **Prep time:** 10 minutes | **Cook time:** 25 minutes

- 16 oz chicken breast, skinless, boneless, sliced
- 2 tablespoons olive oil
- ½ teaspoon Italian seasoning
- 1 onion, sliced
- 1 teaspoon fresh ginger, chopped
- 1 cup bell pepper, sliced
- ½ cup tomatoes, chopped

1. Heat up olive oil in the skillet.
2. Add chicken, Italian seasonings, and ginger. Cook the mixture for 10 minutes.
3. Add all remaining ingredients and stir well.
4. Cook the meal for 15 minutes over the medium heat.

per serving: 216 calories, 24.8g protein, 5.8g carbohydrates, 10.2g fat, 1.3g fiber, 73mg cholesterol, 61mg sodium, 569mg potassium.

Asparagus Chicken Mix

Yield: 4 servings | **Prep time:** 10 minutes | **Cook time:** 25 minutes

- 1-pound chicken breast, skinless, boneless, chopped
- 2 tablespoons avocado oil
- 1 cup asparagus, trimmed and halved
- ½ teaspoon smoked paprika
- 2 cups tomatoes, chopped

1. Heat up a pan with the oil over medium-high heat, add the chicken and asparagus, stir and cook for 5 minutes.
2. All remaining ingredients and cook the meal for 20 minutes over the medium-high heat.

per serving: 162 calories, 25.7g protein, 5.3g carbohydrates, 4g fat, 2.2g fiber, 73mg cholesterol, 63mg sodium, 729mg potassium.

Artichoke Chicken Stew

Yield: 4 servings | **Prep time:** 10 minutes | **Cook time:** 20 minutes

- 2 tablespoons olive oil
- 1 cup spinach, chopped
- 4 artichoke hearts, chopped
- 1-pound chicken breast, chopped
- ½ teaspoon chili flakes
- 1 cup tomatoes, chopped

1. Heat up a pan with the oil over medium-high heat, add chicken and chili flakes, and cook the chicken for 5 minutes per side
2. Add all remaining ingredients and saute the stew for 15 minutes over the medium heat.

per serving: 275 calories, 30g protein, 19.1g carbohydrates, 10.2g fat, 9.5g fiber, 73mg cholesterol, 218mg sodium, 1168mg potassium.

Creamy Turkey

Yield: 4 servings | **Prep time:** 10 minutes | **Cook time:** 25 minutes

- 1 tablespoon olive oil
- 12 oz turkey fillet, chopped
- 2 cups broccoli, chopped
- 1 cup of soy milk
- 1 teaspoon curry powder

1. Heat up a pan with the oil over medium-high heat, add turkey, curry powder, and broccoli. Stir the ingredients for 10 minutes.
2. Then add soy milk and cook the meal for 15 minutes.

per serving: 160 calories, 21g protein, 7.2g carbohydrates, 5.2g fat, 1.7g fiber, 44mg cholesterol, 239mg sodium, 224mg potassium.

Pumpkin Chicken

Yield: 4 servings | **Prep time:** 10 minutes | **Cook time:** 25 minutes

- 1 pound chicken breasts, skinless, boneless, chopped
- 2 cups of water
- 1 tablespoon sesame oil
- 1 cup butternut squash, chopped
- 1 teaspoon cayenne pepper

1. Heat up a pan with the oil over medium-high heat, add the chicken and cook for 5 minutes.
2. Add all remaining ingredients and cook the meal for 20 minutes.

per serving: 263 calories, 33.2g protein, 4.3g carbohydrates, 11.9g fat, 0.8g fiber, 101mg

cholesterol, 103mg sodium, 409mg potassium.

Chicken with Zucchini Cubes

Yield: 4 servings | **Prep time:** 10 minutes | **Cook time:** 30 minutes
- 1-pound chicken breasts, skinless, boneless, chopped
- 1 cup of water
- 2 zucchinis, roughly cubed
- 1 tablespoon olive oil
- 1 cup tomatoes, chopped
- 1 yellow onion, chopped
- 1 teaspoon chili powder

1. Heat up a pan with the oil over medium-high heat, add the chicken and the onion, toss and brown for 5 minutes.
2. Add all remaining ingredients, stir well and cook for 25 minutes more.

per serving: 282 calories, 34.8g protein, 8g carbohydrates, 12.3g fat, 2.4g fiber, 101mg cholesterol, 119mg sodium, 692mg potassium.

Chicken Dill Soup

Yield: 5 servings | **Prep time:** 10 minutes | **Cook time:** 45 minutes
- 1-pound chicken breast, skinless, boneless, chopped
- 1 cup carrot, shredded
- 5 cups of water
- 1 cup yellow onion, chopped
- 1 teaspoon smoked paprika
- ½ teaspoon chili powder
- ½ cup fresh dill, chopped

1. Put the chicken in a pot.
2. Add all remaining ingredients except dill and cook the soup over the medium heat for 40 minutes.

per serving: 136 calories, 20.7g protein, 7.4g carbohydrates, 2.6g fat, 1.9g fiber, 58mg cholesterol, 82mg sodium, 616mg potassium.

Avocado Chicken Slices

Yield: 4 servings | **Prep time:** 10 minutes | **Cook time:** 30 minutes
- 2 chicken breasts, skinless, boneless, sliced
- 1 tablespoon lemon juice
- 2 tablespoons olive oil
- 1 teaspoon minced garlic
- ½ cup of water
- 1 avocado, peeled, pitted and cut into wedges
- ½ teaspoon cayenne pepper

1. Heat up a pan with the oil over medium heat, add the garlic and the chicken and brown it for 2 minutes on each side.
2. Add all remaining ingredients except avocado and cook the chicken for 25 minutes.
3. Top the chicken with avocado and transfer in the serving plates.

per serving: 285 calories, 27.1g protein, 4.8g carbohydrates, 18.4g fat, 3.5g fiber, 65mg cholesterol, 80mg sodium, 256mg potassium.

Chicken with Collard Greens

Yield: 4 servings | **Prep time:** 10 minutes | **Cook time:** 25 minutes
- 4 cups of water
- 1 onion, chopped
- 1-pound chicken breast, skinless, boneless, chopped
- 2 cups collard greens, chopped
- 1 teaspoon ground black pepper
- ½ teaspoon turmeric
- ½ teaspoon smoked paprika

1. Put all ingredients in the saucepan and close the lid.
2. Cook the meal over the medium heat for 25 minutes.

per serving: 150 calories, 25g protein, 4.5g carbohydrates, 3.1g fat, 1.6g fiber, 73mg cholesterol, 70mg sodium, 482mg potassium.

Turkey with Bok Choy

Yield: 4 servings | **Prep time:** 10 minutes | **Cook time:** 25 minutes
- 8 oz turkey fillet, sliced
- 2 tablespoons chives, chopped
- 1 pound bok choy, chopped
- 2 tablespoons olive oil
- 1 teaspoon minced ginger
- ½ cup of water

1. Heat up olive oil in the skillet.
2. Add turkey and minced ginger, and roast the ingredients for 5 minutes.
3. Then add water and chives, close the lid, and cook the meal for 15 minutes.
4. Add bok choy, stir well, and cook the meal for 5 minutes more.

per serving: 130 calories, 13.6g protein, 2.9g carbohydrates, 7.5g fat, 1.2g fiber, 29mg cholesterol, 203mg sodium, 297mg potassium.

Chili Turkey Fillet

Yield: 4 servings | **Prep time:** 5 minutes | **Cook time:** 40 minutes
- *12 oz turkey fillet, chopped*
- *1 cup low-fat milk*
- *2 cups asparagus, chopped*
- *1 teaspoon chili powder*
- *2 tablespoons olive oil*
- *½ teaspoon cayenne pepper*

1. Heat up a pan with the oil over medium-high heat, add the turkey and cayenne pepper, toss and cook for 5 minutes.
2. Add all remaining ingredients and cook the meal over the medium heat for 35 minutes.

per serving: 182 calories, 21.3g protein, 6.1g carbohydrates, 8.2g fat, 1.7g fiber, 47mg cholesterol, 227mg sodium, 244mg potassium.

Chicken Topped with Coconut

Yield: 8 servings | **Prep time:** 10 minutes | **Cook time:** 50 minutes
- *3 tablespoons olive oil*
- *8 chicken thighs, skinless, boneless*
- *½ teaspoon ground black pepper*
- *1 teaspoon garlic powder*
- *1 cup low-fat yogurt*
- *1 tablespoon coconut shred*

1. Heat up olive oil in the saucepan.
2. Add chicken thighs and sprinkle them with ground black pepper and garlic powder.
3. Cook the chicken for 5 minutes per side.
4. Add yogurt and coconut shred. Close the lid and simmer the meal for 40 minutes over the low heat.

per serving: 350 calories, 44.1g protein, 3.2g carbohydrates, 16.6g fat, 0.1g fiber, 132mg cholesterol, 175mg sodium, 432mg potassium.

Chicken with Red Onion

Yield: 4 servings | **Prep time:** 10 minutes | **Cook time:** 30 minutes
- *1-pound chicken breasts, skinless, boneless, roughly cubed*
- *3 red onions, sliced*
- *2 tablespoons olive oil*
- *1 cup of water*
- *1 teaspoon dried thyme*

1. Heat up a pan with the oil over medium heat, add the onions and sauté for 10 minutes stirring often.
2. Add the chicken and cook for 3 minutes more.
3. Then add water, thyme, and stir the meal well.
4. Cook it for 15 minutes more.

per serving: 223 calories, 25g protein, 7.9g carbohydrates, 9.9g fat, 1.9g fiber, 73mg cholesterol, 63mg sodium, 543mg potassium.

Clove Chicken

Yield: 4 servings | **Prep time:** 10 minutes | **Cook time:** 25 minutes
- *1-pound chicken fillet, sliced*
- *1 teaspoon ground clove*
- *1 tablespoon avocado oil*
- *½ cup tomato, chopped*
- *¼ cup of water*

5. Heat up oil in the saucepan.
6. Add chicken and ground clove and stir the meal for 10 minutes.
7. After this, add tomato and water.
8. Close the lid and simmer the meal for 15 minutes more.

per serving: 226 calories, 33.1g protein, 1.4g carbohydrates, 9g fat, 0.6g fiber, 101mg cholesterol, 100mg sodium, 346mg potassium.

Rice with Turkey

Yield: 4 servings | **Prep time:** 10 minutes | **Cook time:** 25 minutes
- *1-pound turkey fillet, chopped*
- *1 cup wild rice*
- *2 cup of water*
- *1 teaspoon chili powder*
- *2 garlic cloves, minced*
- *2 tablespoons olive oil*
- *1 tablespoon low-fat yogurt*

1. Heat up a pan with the oil over medium heat, add turkey and chili powder.
2. Cook the ingredients for 5 minutes.

3. After this, add all remaining ingredients, stir well, and close the lid.
4. Cook the meal for 40 minutes over the low heat.

per serving: 343 calories, 27.2g protein, 38.1g carbohydrates, 8g fat, 0.9g fiber, 59mg cholesterol, 272mg sodium, 82mg potassium.

Apple Chicken

Yield: 4 servings | **Prep time:** 10 minutes | **Cook time:** 40 minutes

- 4 chicken thighs, skinless, boneless
- ½ teaspoon ground black pepper
- 1 cup apples, chopped
- ½ cup apple juice
- 1 teaspoon margarine

1. Heat up margarine in the saucepan.
2. Add chicken and roast it for 5 minutes per side.
3. After this, add all remaining ingredients and close the lid.
4. Simmer the chicken for 30 minutes.

per serving: 330 calories, 42.5g protein, 11.4g carbohydrates, 11.9g fat, 1.5g fiber, 130mg cholesterol, 139mg sodium, 449mg potassium.

Turkey and Savoy Cabbage Mix

Yield: 4 servings | **Prep time:** 10 minutes | **Cook time:** 30 minutes

- 10 oz turkey fillet, sliced
- 1 cup of water
- 1 tablespoon olive oil
- 1 cup Savoy cabbage, shredded
- 1 teaspoon chili powder
- 1 tablespoon margarine

1. Put all ingredients in the baking pan and cover with the foil.
2. Bake the meal for 30 minutes at 385F.

per serving: 129 calories, 15g protein, 1.4g carbohydrates, 6.8g fat, 0.7g fiber, 37mg cholesterol, 205mg sodium, 44mg potassium.

Soft Sage Turkey

Yield: 4 servings | **Prep time:** 10 minutes | **Cook time:** 35 minutes

- 1-pound turkey fillet, chopped
- 1 tablespoon margarine, melted
- 1 teaspoon dried sage
- 1 tablespoon olive oil

1. Mix up olive oil, margarine, and sage in the shallow bowl.
2. Mix up turkey fillet and oil mixture together, and transfer in the baking pan.
3. Bake the meal at 375F for 35 minutes.

per serving: 163 calories, 23.6g protein, 0.1g carbohydrates, 6.9g fat, 0.1g fiber, 59mg cholesterol, 290mg sodium, 3mg potassium.

Thai Style Chicken Cubes

Yield: 6 servings | **Prep time:** 10 minutes | **Cook time:** 35 minutes

- 16 oz chicken fillet, cubed
- 1 tablespoon scallions, chopped
- ½ cup Thai chili sauce

1. Heat up a pan over medium-high heat, add chicken and roast it for 5 minutes on each side, transfer to a baking dish, add chili sauce and scallions, toss well and transfer the meal in the preheated to 390F oven.
2. Bake the meal for 35 minutes.

per serving: 145 calories, 21.9g protein, 0.3g carbohydrates, 5.6g fat, 0g fiber, 67mg cholesterol, 70mg sodium, 186mg potassium.

Ginger Sauce Chicken

Yield: 4 servings | **Prep time:** 10 minutes | **Cook time:** 35 minutes

- 1 pound chicken breast, skinless, boneless, chopped
- 1 tablespoon ginger, grated
- 1 tablespoon olive oil
- 1 teaspoon minced garlic
- 1 teaspoon smoked paprika
- ¼ cup low-fat yogurt

1. Heat up olive oil in the skillet. Add chicken and cook it for 5 minutes per side.
2. Then add ginger, minced garlic, and smoked paprika.
3. Stir the chicken well and add yogurt.
4. Close the lid and cook the meal for 25 minutes.

per serving: 177 calories, 25.2g protein, 2.6g carbohydrates, 6.7g fat, 0.4g fiber, 74mg cholesterol, 69mg sodium, 489mg potassium.

Quinoa Chicken

Yield: 6 servings | **Prep time:** 10 minutes | **Cook time:** 30 minutes

- *1-pound chicken breast, skinless, boneless, chopped*
- *1 tablespoon avocado oil*
- *1 cup quinoa*
- *2 cups of water*
- *1 tablespoon lemon juice*
- *1 tablespoon dill, chopped*
- *½ teaspoon ground black pepper*
- *1 tablespoon red curry paste*

1. Heat up a pan with the oil over medium-high heat, add the chicken and brown it for 10 minutes.
2. Add all remaining ingredients and stir the mixture until homogenous.
3. Close the lid and simmer the chicken for 20 minutes over the medium-high heat.

per serving: 206 calories, 20.2g protein, 19.3g carbohydrates, 4.7g fat, 2.2g fiber, 48mg cholesterol, 174mg sodium, 470mg potassium.

Parsnip Turkey

Yield: 4 servings | **Prep time:** 10 minutes | **Cook time:** 25 minutes

- *12 oz turkey fillet, sliced*
- *2 parsnips, chopped*
- *1 tablespoon parsley, chopped*
- *2 tablespoons sesame oil*
- *1 onion, chopped*
- *1 cup of water*

1. Heat up a pan with the oil over medium heat, add the onion and sauté for 5 minutes.
2. Add the turkey, toss and cook for 5 minutes more.
3. Add all remaining ingredients, close the lid and simmer the meal for 15 minutes.

per serving: 177 calories, 18.4g protein, 8.6g carbohydrates, 7.3g fat, 2.3g fiber, 44mg cholesterol, 199mg sodium, 171mg potassium.

Chopped Chicken

Yield: 4 servings | **Prep time:** 10 minutes | **Cook time:** 25 minutes

- 1 teaspoon ground paprika
- 1 teaspoon tomato paste
- 1 tablespoon olive oil
- 1-pound chicken fillet, chopped

1. Mix up all ingredients in the baking pan and cover with foil.
2. Bake the chopped chicken for 30 minutes at 375F.

per serving: 248 calories, 33g protein, 0.6g carbohydrates, 12g fat, 0.3g fiber, 101mg cholesterol, 99mg sodium, 301mg potassium.

Chicken in Bell Pepper

Yield: 5 servings | **Prep time:** 10 minutes | **Cook time:** 35 minutes

- *16 oz chicken breast, skinless, boneless, chopped*
- *2 cups bell pepper, chopped*
- *1 teaspoon dried thyme*
- *1 teaspoon smoked paprika*
- *1 teaspoon ground black pepper*
- *1 teaspoon dried oregano*
- *1 cup low-fat yogurt*

1. Mix up all ingredients in the baking pan and flatten well.
2. Bake the chicken for 35 minutes at 375F.

per serving: 157 calories, 22.7g protein, 7.9g carbohydrates, 3.1g fat, 1.1g fiber, 61mg cholesterol, 82mg sodium, 562mg potassium.

Chickpea Chicken

Yield: 4 servings | **Prep time:** 10 minutes | **Cook time:** 25 minutes

- *1 cup chickpeas, cooked*
- *½ cup of water*
- *1-pound chicken breast, skinless, boneless, chopped*
- *1 teaspoon ground black pepper*
- *1 teaspoon oregano, dried*
- *1 teaspoon nutmeg, ground*
- *1 tablespoon margarine*

1. Heat up margarine in the saucepan and add chicken breast, ground black pepper, oregano, and nutmeg.
2. Roast the chicken for 10 minutes.
3. Then stir well, and add water and chickpeas.
4. Close the lid and cook the meal for 15 minutes more.

per serving: 342 calories, 33.9g protein, 31.2g carbohydrates, 9g fat, 9.1g fiber, 73mg cholesterol, 105mg sodium, 874mg potassium.

Carrot Chicken

Yield: 8 servings | **Prep time:** 10 minutes | **Cook time:** 60 minutes
- 2 onions, chopped
- 8 chicken thighs, skinless, boneless
- 1 teaspoon minced garlic
- 1 tablespoon margarine
- ½ teaspoon chili flakes
- 1 cup of water
- 1 cup carrot, shredded

1. Melt margarine in the saucepan and add the onion. Cook it for 5 minutes.
2. Then add all remaining ingredients and stir the mixture well.
3. Cook it with the closed lid for 55 minutes over the low heat.

per serving: 307 calories, 42.7g protein, 4.1g carbohydrates, 12.3g fat, 0.9g fiber, 130mg cholesterol, 154mg sodium, 442mg potassium.

Turkey with Olives

Yield: 4 servings | **Prep time:** 10 minutes | **Cook time:** 35 minutes
- 1 cup green olives, pitted and halved
- 1 pound turkey fillet, sliced
- 1 tablespoon parsley, chopped
- 1 cup tomato puree
- 1 tablespoon olive oil

1. Grease a baking dish with the oil.
2. Add all remaining ingredients in the baking pan, flatten well, and cover with foil.
3. Bake the meal ta 385F for 35 minutes.

per serving: 200 calories, 24.9g protein, 7.8g carbohydrates, 7.8g fat, 2.3g fiber, 59mg cholesterol, 568mg sodium, 282mg potassium.

Chicken Tomato Mix

Yield: 4 servings | **Prep time:** 10 minutes | **Cook time:** 30 minutes
- 1-pound chicken breast, skinless, boneless, chopped
- 1 cup tomatoes, chopped
- 1 chili pepper
- 1 tablespoon margarine
- ¼ cup of water

1. Heat up margarine and add chili pepper. Roast it for 2 minutes.
2. Add chicken breast and stir the mixture well. Cook it for 8 minutes.
3. Then add tomatoes and water.
4. Close the lid and cook the meal for 20 minutes.

per serving: 163 calories, 24.5g protein, 1.9g carbohydrates, 5.8g fat, 0.6g fiber, 73mg cholesterol, 94mg sodium, 530mg potassium.

5-Spices Chicken Wings

Yield: 4 servings | **Prep time:** 10 minutes | **Cook time:** 30 minutes
- 1-pound chicken wings, skinless, boneless
- 1 tablespoon five-spices
- 2 tablespoons margarine, melted

5. Rub the chicken wings with condiments and sprinkle with margarine.
6. Bake the chicken wings for 30 minutes at 365F.

per serving: 272 calories, 32.9g protein, 1.6g carbohydrates, 14.1g fat, 0g fiber, 101mg cholesterol, 195mg sodium, 279mg potassium.

Onion and Curry Paste Chicken

Yield: 6 servings | **Prep time:** 10 minutes | **Cook time:** 30 minutes
- 1 yellow onion, chopped
- 3 garlic cloves, minced
- 1 tablespoon olive oil
- 1 teaspoon curry paste
- 1-pound chicken breast, skinless, boneless
- 2 cups low-fat yogurt
- ½ cup fresh cilantro, chopped

1. Heat up olive oil in the saucepan.
2. Add yogurt, cilantro, curry paste, garlic, and onion.
3. Simmer the mixture for 5 minutes.
4. Then add chopped chicken and stir the mixture well.
5. Cook it for 25 minutes over the medium heat.

per serving: 180 calories, 21.1g protein, 8.3g carbohydrates, 5.8g fat, 0.5g fiber, 53mg cholesterol, 97mg sodium, 511mg potassium.

Cumin Chicken Thighs

Yield: 4 servings | **Prep time:** 10 minutes | **Cook time:** 30 minutes
- 1 red onion, chopped
- 4 chicken thighs, skinless, boneless
- 1 cup cauliflower, chopped

- *1 teaspoon cumin seeds*
- *1 cup low-fat milk*
- *1 teaspoon garlic powder*
- *1 tablespoon margarine*

1. Melt margarine and add chicken thighs.
2. Cook the meat for 5 minutes per side.
3. Add all remaining ingredients and stir gently.
4. Close the lid and cook the meal for 25 minutes over the medium heat.

per serving: 350 calories, 45.3g protein, 7.7g carbohydrates, 14.4g fat, 1.4g fiber, 133mg cholesterol, 195mg sodium, 581mg potassium.

Beef and Pork

Herbs de Provence Pork Chops

Yield: 4 servings | **Prep time:** 15 minutes | **Cook time:** 14 minutes
- 4 pork top loin chops
- 1 tablespoon herbs de Provence
- 4 teaspoons olive oil

1. Tub the pork chops with herbs de Provence and sprinkle with olive oil.
2. After this, preheat the grill to 390F.
3. Put the pork chops in the grill and roast them for 7 minutes per side.

per serving: 231 calories, 25.9g protein, 0g carbohydrates, 13.6g fat, 0g fiber, 65mg cholesterol, 48mg sodium, 425mg potassium.

Curry Pork Chops

Yield: 2 servings | **Prep time:** 10 minutes | **Cook time:** 25 minutes
- 2 pork loin chops
- 1 teaspoon curry powder
- ¼ cup of soy milk
- 1 onion, diced
- 1 tablespoon olive oil

1. Heat up olive oil in the skillet.
2. Add pork chops and roast them for 5 minutes per side.
3. Remove the meat from the skillet and add diced onion. Cook it for 4 minutes or until the onion is tender.
4. Then add curry powder and soy milk.
5. Bring the mixture to boil.
6. Add cooked pork chops and coat them in the curry mixture well.
7. Close the lid and simmer the meal for 10 minutes on low heat.

per serving: 358 calories, 19.7g protein, 7.6g carbohydrates, 27.6g fat, 1.7g fiber, 69mg cholesterol, 74mg sodium, 407mg potassium.

Pork Roast with Orange Sauce

Yield: 4 servings | **Prep time:** 15 minutes | **Cook time:** 80 minutes
- 1-pound pork loin roast
- ½ cup carrot, diced
- ½ cup celery stalk, chopped
- ½ cup onion, diced
- 1 teaspoon Italian seasonings
- 1 cup of orange juice
- 1 tablespoon potato starch

1. Rub the pork loin roast with Italian seasonings.
2. Then put the carrot, celery stalk, and diced onion in the tray.
3. Put the meat over the vegetables. Add orange juice.
4. Bake the meat for 75 minutes at 365F.
5. After this, transfer all vegetables and juice in the saucepan and bring it to boil.
6. Blend the mixture with the help of the blender. Add potato starch and whisk it well.
7. Simmer the sauce for 2 minutes.
8. Slice the cooked meat and sprinkle it with orange sauce.

per serving: 292 calories, 33.2g protein, 12.2g carbohydrates, 11.4g fat, 1g fiber, 93mg cholesterol, 87mg sodium, 704mg potassium.

Southwestern Steak

Yield: 2 servings | **Prep time:** 15 minutes | **Cook time:** 16 minutes
- 2 beef flank steaks
- 1 tablespoon lemon juice
- 1 teaspoon chili flakes
- 1 teaspoon garlic powder
- 1 tablespoon avocado oil

1. Preheat the grill to 385F.
2. Then rub the meat with chili flakes and garlic powder.
3. Then sprinkle it with lemon juice and avocado oil.
4. Grill the steaks for 8 minutes per side.

per serving: 174 calories, 26.2g protein, 1.6g carbohydrates, 6.3g fat, 0.5g fiber, 76mg cholesterol, 58mg sodium, 392mg potassium.

Tender Pork Medallions

Yield: 3 servings | **Prep time:** 10 minutes | **Cook time:** 25 minutes
- 12 oz pork tenderloin
- 1 teaspoon dried sage
- 1 tablespoon margarine
- 1 teaspoon ground black pepper
- ½ cup low-fat yogurt

1. Cut the pork tenderloin into 3 medallions and sprinkle with sage and ground black pepper.

2. Heat up margarine in the saucepan and add pork medallions.
3. Roast them for 5 minutes per side.
4. Then add yogurt and coat the meat in it well.
5. Close the lid and simmer the medallions for 15 minutes over the medium heat.
per serving: 227 calories, 32.4g protein, 3.5g carbohydrates, 8.3g fat, 0.3g fiber, 85mg cholesterol, 138mg sodium, 586mg potassium.

Garlic Pork Meatballs

Yield: 2 servings | **Prep time:** 10 minutes | **Cook time:** 28 minutes
- 2 pork medallions
- 1 teaspoon minced garlic
- ¼ cup of coconut milk
- 1 tablespoon olive oil
- 1 teaspoon cayenne pepper

1. Sprinkle each pork medallion with cayenne pepper.
2. Heat up olive oil in the skillet and add meat.
3. Roast the pork medallions for 3 minutes from each side.
4. After this, add coconut milk and minced garlic. Close the lid and simmer the meat for 20 minutes on low heat.
per serving: 284 calories, 25.9g protein, 2.6g carbohydrates, 18.8g fat, 0.9g fiber, 70mg cholesterol, 60mg sodium, 103mg potassium.

Fajita Pork Strips

Yield: 4 servings | **Prep time:** 10 minutes | **Cook time:** 35 minutes
- 16 oz pork sirloin
- 1 tablespoon Fajita seasonings
- 1 tablespoon canola oil

1. Cut the pork sirloin into the strips and sprinkle with fajita seasonings and canola oil.
2. Then transfer the meat in the baking tray in one layer.
3. Bake it for 35 minutes at 365F. Stir the meat every 10 minutes during cooking.
per serving: 184 calories, 18.5g protein, 1.3g carbohydrates, 10.8g fat, 0g fiber, 64mg cholesterol, 157mg sodium, 0mg potassium.

Pepper Pork Tenderloins

Yield: 2 servings | **Prep time:** 15 minutes | **Cook time:** 60 minutes
- 8 oz pork tenderloin
- 1 tablespoon mustard
- 1 teaspoon ground black pepper
- 2 tablespoons olive oil

1. Rub the meat with mustard and sprinkle with ground black pepper.
2. Then brush it with olive oil and wrap in the foil.
3. Bake the meat for 60 minutes at 375F.
4. Then discard the foil and slice the tenderloin into servings.
per serving: 311 calories, 31.2g protein, 2.6g carbohydrates, 19.6g fat, 1.1g fiber, 83mg cholesterol, 65mg sodium, 529mg potassium.

Spiced Beef

Yield: 4 servings | **Prep time:** 10 minutes | **Cook time:** 80 minutes
- 1-pound beef sirloin
- 1 tablespoon five-spice seasoning
- 1 bay leaf
- 2 cups of water
- 1 teaspoon peppercorn

1. Rub the meat with five-spice seasoning and put in the saucepan.
2. Add nay leaf, water, and peppercorns.
3. Close the lid and simmer it for 80 minutes on the medium heat.
4. Chop the cooked meat and sprinkle it with hot spiced water from the saucepan.
per serving: 213 calories, 34.5g protein, 0.5g carbohydrates, 7.1g fat, 0.2g fiber, 101mg cholesterol, 116mg sodium, 466mg potassium.

Tomato Beef

Yield: 2 servings | **Prep time:** 10 minutes | **Cook time:** 17 minutes
- 2 chuck shoulder steaks
- ¼ cup tomato sauce
- 1 tablespoon olive oil

1. Brush the steaks with tomato sauce and olive oil and transfer in the preheated to 390F grill.
2. Grill the meat for 9 minutes.
3. Then flip it on another side and cook for 8 minutes more.
per serving: 247 calories, 21.4g protein, 1.7g carbohydrates, 17.1g fat, 0.5g fiber, 70mg

cholesterol, 231mg sodium, 101mg potassium.

Hoisin Pork

Yield: 4 servings | **Prep time:** 10 minutes | **Cook time:** 14 minutes
- 1-pound pork loin steaks
- 2 tablespoons hoisin sauce
- 1 tablespoon apple cider vinegar
- 1 teaspoon olive oil

1. Rub the pork steaks with hoisin sauce, apple cider vinegar, and olive oil.
2. Then preheat the grill to 395F.
3. Put the pork steak in the grill and cook them for 7 minutes per side.

per serving: 263 calories, 39.3g protein, 3.6g carbohydrates, 10.1g fat, 0.2g fiber, 0mg cholesterol, 130mg sodium, 12mg potassium.

Sage Beef Loin

Yield: 2 servings | **Prep time:** 10 minutes | **Cook time:** 18 minutes
- 10 oz beef loin, strips
- 1 garlic clove, diced
- 2 tablespoons margarine
- 1 teaspoon dried sage

1. Toss margarine in the skillet.
2. Add garlic and dried sage and roast them for 2 minutes on low heat.
3. Add beef loin strips and roast them for 15 minutes on medium heat. Stir the meat occasionally.

per serving: 363 calories, 38.2g protein, 0.8g carbohydrates, 23.2g fat, 0.2g fiber, 101mg cholesterol, 211mg sodium, 497mg potassium.

Beef Chili

Yield: 4 servings | **Prep time:** 10 minutes | **Cook time:** 30 minutes
- 1 cup lean lean ground beef
- 1 onion, diced
- 1 tablespoon olive oil
- 1 cup crushed tomatoes
- ½ cup red kidney beans, cooked
- ½ cup of water
- 1 teaspoon chili seasonings

1. Heat up olive oil in the saucepan and add lean ground beef.
2. Cook it for 7 minutes over the medium heat.
3. Then add chili seasonings and diced onion. Stir the ingredients and cook them for 10 minutes.
4. After this, add water, crushed tomatoes, red kidney beans, and stir the chili well.
5. Close the lid and simmer the meal for 13 minutes.

per serving: 220 calories, 18.3g protein, 22g carbohydrates, 6.7g fat, 6.1g fiber, 34mg cholesterol, 177mg sodium, 530mg potassium.

Celery Beef Stew

Yield: 6 servings | **Prep time:** 5 minutes | **Cook time:** 55 minutes
- 1-pound beef loin, chopped
- 2 cups celery stalk, chopped
- 1 garlic clove, diced
- 1 yellow onion, diced
- 1 tablespoon olive oil
- 1 tablespoon tomato paste
- 1 teaspoon chili powder
- 1 teaspoon dried dill
- 2 cups of water

1. Roast the beef loin with olive oil in the saucepan for 5 minutes.
2. After this, add all remaining ingredients and close the lid.
3. Cook the stew for 50 minutes on medium heat,

per serving: 150 calories, 14.6g protein, 4.6g carbohydrates, 7.9g fat, 1.2g fiber, 41mg cholesterol, 370mg sodium, 158mg potassium.

Beef Skillet

Yield: 3 servings | **Prep time:** 10 minutes | **Cook time:** 30 minutes
- 1 cup lean lean ground beef
- 1 cup bell pepper, sliced
- 2 tomatoes, chopped
- 1 chili pepper, chopped
- 1 tablespoon olive oil
- ½ cup of water

1. Heat up olive oil in the skillet and add lean ground beef.
2. Roast it for 10 minutes.
3. Then stir the meat well and add chili pepper and bell pepper. Roast the ingredients for 10 minutes more.
4. Add tomatoes and water.

5. Close the lid and simmer the meal for 10 minutes.
per serving: 167 calories, 16.1g protein, 6.3g carbohydrates, 8.8g fat, 1.6g fiber, 46mg cholesterol, 50mg sodium, 508mg potassium.

Hot Beef Strips

Yield: 3 servings | **Prep time:** 10 minutes | **Cook time:** 15 minutes
- 9 oz beef tenders
- 2 tablespoons cayenne pepper
- 1 tablespoon lemon juice
- 2 tablespoons canola oil

1. Cut the beef tenders into the strips and rub with cayenne pepper.
2. Sprinkle the meat with lemon juice and put it in the hot skillet.
3. Add canola oil and roast the meat for 15 minutes on medium heat. Stir it from time to time to avoid burning.

per serving: 231 calories, 22.5g protein, 2.1g carbohydrates, 14.6g fat, 1g fiber, 54mg cholesterol, 62mg sodium, 327mg potassium.

Ground Turkey Fiesta

Yield: 2 servings | **Prep time:** 10 minutes | **Cook time:** 20 minutes
- ½ cup ground turkey
- ½ cup white beans, cooked
- ½ cup corn kernels, cooked
- 1 tablespoon olive oil
- 1 teaspoon dried rosemary
- 1 teaspoon cayenne pepper
- ½ cup tomato puree

1. Put ground turkey in the skillet.
2. Add olive oil, cayenne pepper, and dried rosemary.
3. Cook the ingredients for 10 minutes.
4. Then stir them well and add white beans, corn kernels, and tomato puree.
5. Close the lid and cook the meal for 10 minutes on the low heat.

per serving: 352 calories, 27.4g protein, 44.2g carbohydrates, 9.4g fat, 10.4g fiber, 31mg cholesterol, 60mg sodium, 1474mg potassium.

Sloppy Joe

Yield: 4 servings | **Prep time:** 10 minutes | **Cook time:** 35 minutes
- 1 cup lean ground beef
- 1 cup onion, diced
- ½ cup sweet peppers, diced
- 1 teaspoon minced garlic
- 1 tablespoon canola oil
- 1 teaspoon liquid honey
- ½ cup tomato puree
- 1 teaspoon tomato paste

1. Mix up canola oil and lean ground beef in the saucepan.
2. Add onion and sweet pepper and stir the ingredient well.
3. Cook them for 10 minutes.
4. Then add honey, tomato puree, and tomato paste. Mix up the mixture well.
5. Close the lid and cook it for 25 minutes on medium heat.

per serving: 134 calories, 7.6g protein, 8.7g carbohydrates, 7.7g fat, 1.9g fiber, 22mg cholesterol, 34mg sodium, 170mg potassium.

Turmeric Meatloaf

Yield: 6 servings | **Prep time:** 15 minutes | **Cook time:** 50 minutes
- 1 teaspoon ground turmeric
- 1 teaspoon chili flakes
- 2 oz minced onion
- 2 cups lean ground beef
- 2 tablespoons semolina
- 1 tablespoon ketchup
- 1 egg, beaten
- 1 teaspoon olive oil

1. Brush the meatloaf mold with olive oil.
2. Then in the mixing bowl, mix up all ingredients from the list above.
3. Transfer the meat mixture in the prepared meatloaf and flatten it well.
4. Bake the meatloaf at 375F for 50 minutes.
5. Then cool it well and slice into servings.

per serving: 136 calories, 16.5g protein, 4.4g carbohydrates, 5.5g fat, 0.4g fiber, 73mg cholesterol, 82mg sodium, 285mg potassium.

Beef Casserole

Yield: 5 servings | **Prep time:** 15 minutes | **Cook time:** 45 minutes
- 1 cup zucchini, grated
- 1 teaspoon margarine
- 8 oz lean ground beef
- 1 bell pepper, chopped
- 1 cup tomatoes, crushed

- 1 teaspoon dried thyme
- 1 teaspoon ground black pepper
- 4 oz low-fat feta, crumbled
1. Grease the casserole mold with margarine.
2. Mix up ground black pepper, dried thyme, and lean ground beef together.
3. Put the mixture in the casserole mold and flatten well.
4. Top it with zucchini, bell pepper, and crumbled low-fat feta.
5. Add crushed tomatoes and cover with foil.
6. Bake the beef casserole in the preheated to 385F oven for 45 minutes.

per serving: 164 calories,18.9g protein, 5.6g carbohydrates, 8g fat, 1.6g fiber, 8mg cholesterol, 56mg sodium, 379mg potassium.

Garlic Steak

Yield: 2 servings | **Prep time:** 10 minutes | **Cook time:** 25 minutes
- 2 lean beef steaks
- 1 teaspoon minced garlic
- 1 tablespoon olive oil
- 1 teaspoon apple cider vinegar
1. Rub the meat with minced garlic and sprinkle with apple cider vinegar.
2. Then heat up skillet well and add olive oil.
3. Add prepared beef steaks and roast them on medium heat for 10 minutes per side.

per serving: 221 calories,25.9g protein, 0.5g carbohydrates, 12.3g fat, 0g fiber, 76mg cholesterol, 56mg sodium, 350mg potassium.

Ham Casserole

Yield: 4 servings | **Prep time:** 15 minutes | **Cook time:** 40 minutes
- 8 oz low-sodium ham, chopped
- ¼ cup low-fat yogurt
- 1 teaspoon Italian seasonings
- ½ cup red kidney beans, cooked
- 1 cup spinach, chopped
- ¼ cup low-sodium vegetable broth
1. Mix up yogurt and ham. Add Italian seasonings.
2. Then transfer the mixture in the casserole mold.
3. Top it with spinach and red kidney beans.
4. Then add vegetable broth and cover the casserole with foil.
5. Bake it for 40 minutes at 365F.

per serving: 117 calories,10.1g protein, 16.4g carbohydrates, 1.2g fat, 3.7g fiber, 11mg cholesterol, 197mg sodium, 438mg potassium.

Beef Ranch Steak

Yield: 2 servings | **Prep time:** 10 minutes | **Cook time:** 16 minutes
- 8 oz beef ranch steak (2 servings)
- 1 teaspoon mustard
- 1 tablespoon olive oil
- ½ teaspoon ground nutmeg
1. Mix up mustard, olive oil, and ground nutmeg.
2. Then brush the meat with mustard mixture and transfer in the preheated to 400F grill.
3. Grill the meat for 8 minutes per side.
4. Then slice the steaks.

per serving: 465 calories,23.2g protein, 35.5g carbohydrates, 25g fat, 4.2g fiber, 0mg cholesterol, 0mg sodium, 13mg potassium.

Pork Casserole

Yield: 4 servings | **Prep time:** 15 minutes | **Cook time:** 30 minutes
- ¼ cup of rice, cooked
- 10 oz pork loin, chopped
- 4 tomatoes, chopped
- 1 chili pepper, chopped
- ½ tablespoon olive oil
1. Roast the pork loin, chili pepper, and olive oil in the skillet for 10 minutes.
2. Then transfer the ingredients in the casserole mold.
3. Add chopped tomatoes and rice. Mix up the ingredients and cover with foil.
4. Bake the casserole for 20 minutes at 365F.

per serving: 251 calories,21.3g protein, 14.1g carbohydrates, 12g fat, 1.7g fiber, 57mg cholesterol, 51mg sodium, 607mg potassium.

Melted Beef Bites

Yield: 5 servings | **Prep time:** 10 minutes | **Cook time:** 50 minutes
- 1-pound beef tenderloin, chopped
- 2 cups of water
- 1 teaspoon peppercorns

- 1 teaspoon dried rosemary
- 1 tablespoon tomato paste
- 1 teaspoon margarine
1. Toss margarine in the saucepan and melt it.
2. Add chopped beef and roast it for 5 minutes.
3. After this, add peppercorns, rosemary, and tomato paste. Stir well.
4. Add water and close the lid.
5. Cook the meat on medium heat for 50 minutes.

per serving: 180 calories, 27.7g protein, 1g carbohydrates, 6.5g fat, 0.3g fiber, 81mg cholesterol, 75mg sodium, 407mg potassium.

Pork Sliders Meat

Yield: 3 servings | **Prep time:** 10 minutes | **Cook time:** 60 minutes
- 12 oz pork shoulder roast
- 1 teaspoon ground paprika
- 2 tablespoons ketchup
- 1 teaspoon liquid honey
- 1 teaspoon cayenne pepper
- 1 cup of water
- 1 teaspoon olive oil
1. Pour olive oil in the saucepan and heat it up.
2. Add meat and roast it for 5 minutes per side or until the meat is golden brown from each side.
3. Then add all remaining ingredients and close the lid.
4. Cook the meat for 50 minutes.
5. When the meat is tender, shred it with the help of the fork.

per serving: 325 calories, 19.4g protein, 5.2g carbohydrates, 24.9g fat, 0.5g fiber, 80mg cholesterol, 190mg sodium, 69mg potassium.

Beef Saute

Yield: 2 servings | **Prep time:** 10 minutes | **Cook time:** 47 minutes
- 8 oz beef tenderloin, chopped
- 1 tablespoon avocado oil
- 1 chili pepper, chopped
- 2 bell peppers, chopped
- 1 cup tomatoes, chopped
- ¼ cup of water
1. Heat up avocado oil in the deep skillet.
2. Add chili pepper and bell pepper and roast the vegetables for 5 minutes.
3. Then stir them well and add beef. Roast the meat for 10 minutes.
4. Add tomatoes and water.
5. Close the lid and saute the meat for 30 minutes on low heat.

per serving: 298 calories, 34.9g protein, 13.1g carbohydrates, 11.7g fat, 3.1g fiber, 104mg cholesterol, 76mg sodium, 869mg potassium.

Light Shepherd Pie

Yield: 4 servings | **Prep time:** 15 minutes | **Cook time:** 40 minutes
- 1 cup lean ground beef
- 1 teaspoon tomato paste
- 1 teaspoon chili powder
- ½ cup green peas
- 1 cup potatoes, mashed
- ¼ cup low-fat yogurt
- 1 teaspoon olive oil
1. Put lean ground beef in the skillet.
2. Add olive oil and chili powder.
3. Roast the meat for 10 minutes.
4. Then add tomato paste and mix it up.
5. After this, transfer the mixture in the casserole mold.
6. Top it with green peas and mashed potatoes.
7. Flatten the potato well.
8. Then sprinkle it with yogurt and cover with foil.
9. Bake the shepherd pie for 30 minutes at 375F.

per serving: 139 calories, 13.9g protein, 10.2g carbohydrates, 4.5g fat, 2.1g fiber, 35mg cholesterol, 54mg sodium, 435mg potassium.

Meat&Mushrooms Bowl

Yield: 2 servings | **Prep time:** 10 minutes | **Cook time:** 25 minutes
- 6 oz pork sirloin, sliced
- 1 cup cremini mushrooms, sliced
- 1 tablespoon olive oil
- 1 teaspoon dried dill
- 1 teaspoon ground black pepper
- ½ cup low-fat yogurt
1. Roast sliced meat in the skillet for 5 minutes.

2. Then stir it well and add dried dill, ground black pepper, and mushrooms.
3. Cook the ingredients for 10 minutes on medium heat.
4. After this, add yogurt and stir the ingredients well.
5. Close the lid and cook the meal for 10 minutes more.
6. Transfer the cooked meal in the serving bowls.
per serving: 269 calories, 22.1g protein, 6.8g carbohydrates, 16.2g fat, 0.6g fiber, 57mg cholesterol, 92mg sodium, 334mg potassium.

Tandoori Beef

Yield: 2 servings | **Prep time:** 15 minutes | **Cook time:** 30 minutes
- 10 oz beef tenderloin, cubed
- 1 teaspoon garam masala
- 2 bell peppers
- 1 tablespoon olive oil
- 1 tablespoon tomato puree
- 1 tablespoon low-fat yogurt

1. Mix up yogurt, tomato puree, and garam masala.
2. Then coat the beef cubes in the condiment mixture.
3. String the meat and bell peppers one-by-one in the skewers.
4. Bake the tandoori beef for 30 minutes at 375F or until the meat is tender.
per serving: 398 calories, 42.8g protein, 10.2g carbohydrates, 20.4g fat, 1.8g fiber, 131mg cholesterol, 96mg sodium, 782mg potassium.

Oregano Pork Tenderloin

Yield: 4 servings | **Prep time:** 15 minutes | **Cook time:** 60 minutes
- 1-pound pork tenderloin
- 1 tablespoon dried oregano
- 2 tablespoons avocado oil
- 1 teaspoon onion powder
- 1 teaspoon lime zest, grated

1. Rub the pork tenderloin with dried oregano, onion powder, and lime zest.
2. Then brush it with avocado oil and wrap in the foil.
3. Bake the meat at 375F for 60 minutes.
4. Slice the cooked meat into servings.

per serving: 177 calories, 30g protein, 1.7g carbohydrates, 5g fat, 0.9g fiber, 83mg cholesterol, 68mg sodium, 525mg potassium.

Baked Beef Tenders

Yield: 3 servings | **Prep time:** 15 minutes | **Cook time:** 40 minutes
- 12 oz beef tenderloin
- 1 teaspoon dried rosemary
- 1 onion, chopped
- 1 tablespoon avocado oil

1. Cut the meat into the tenders and sprinkle with rosemary and avocado oil.
2. Then transfer it in the lined baking tray. Top the meat with onion and cover with foil.
3. Bake the meat for 30 minutes at 365F.
4. Then shake the meat well and cook it without foil for 10 minutes more.
per serving: 265 calories, 33.3g protein, 3.9g carbohydrates, 11.1g fat, 1.2g fiber, 104mg cholesterol, 69mg sodium, 477mg potassium.

Pork Stuffed Peppers

Yield: 3 servings | **Prep time:** 15 minutes | **Cook time:** 45 minutes
- 3 bell peppers
- 1 cup lean ground pork
- 1 cup crushed tomatoes with juice
- 1 teaspoon ground black pepper
- 2 tablespoons minced onion
- 1 carrot, grated
- ¼ cup low-fat yogurt

1. Mix up lean ground pork, ground black pepper, minced onion, and carrot,
2. Then trim the bell peppers and remove the seeds.
3. Fill the bell peppers with lean ground pork and transfer in the saucepan.
4. Add crushed tomatoes and yogurt.
5. Close the lid and simmer the meal for 45 minutes on medium-low heat.
per serving: 394 calories, 31.3g protein, 716.g carbohydrates, 22.2g fat, 5.5g fiber, 99mg cholesterol, 268mg sodium, 717mg potassium.

White Cabbage Rolls

Yield: 4 servings | **Prep time:** 15 minutes | **Cook time:** 30 minutes
- 4 white cabbage leaves

- ½ cup carrot, grated
- 1 teaspoon Italian seasonings
- ¼ cup tomato puree
- 6 oz lean ground pork

1. In the mixing bowl, mix up Italian seasonings, carrot, and lean ground pork.
2. Then fill the white cabbage leaves with meat mixture to get the cabbage rolls and put in the small casserole mold.
3. Add tomato puree and transfer in the preheated to 365F oven.
4. Cook the cabbage rolls for 30 minutes.

per serving: 80 calories, 11.7g protein, 3.8g carbohydrates, 1.9g fat, 1g fiber, 32mg cholesterol, 41mg sodium, 318mg potassium.

Mandarin Pork Loin

Yield: 4 servings | **Prep time:** 15 minutes | **Cook time:** 45 minutes

- 1-pound pork loin
- 2 mandarins, peeled
- 1 teaspoon ground black pepper
- 1 teaspoon minced garlic
- 1 tablespoon mustard
- 1 tablespoon olive oil

1. Blend together mandarins, ground black pepper, minced garlic, mustard, and olive oil.
2. Then carefully rub the pork loin with the mandarin mixture and transfer the meat in the foil.
3. Add remaining mandarin mixture and wrap the meat.
4. Bake it for 45 minutes at 375F.
5. Then discard the foil and slice the meat.

per serving: 340 calories, 32.3g protein, 6.6g carbohydrates, 20.2g fat, 1.1g fiber, 91mg cholesterol, 72mg sodium, 571mg potassium.

Beef Stroganoff Strips

Yield: 2 servings | **Prep time:** 10 minutes | **Cook time:** 20 minutes

- 1 teaspoon ground black pepper
- 1 teaspoon dried dill
- 1 tablespoon potato starch
- ½ cup low-fat milk
- 1 teaspoon olive oil
- 8 oz beef round steak

1. Cut the beef into the strips and sprinkle with ground black pepper and dill.
2. Then transfer the strips in the skillet. Add olive oil.
3. Roast the meat for 4 minutes per side.
4. After this, add milk and bring the mixture to boil.
5. Add potato starch and stir it. Simmer the meat until thicken.

per serving: 313 calories, 38.2g protein, 9g carbohydrates, 13g fat, 0.4g fiber, 98mg cholesterol, 98mg sodium, 622mg potassium.

Spinach Pork Cubes

Yield: 4 servings | **Prep time:** 10 minutes | **Cook time:** 12 minutes

- 4 pork loin chops, cubed
- 4 teaspoons spinach, blended

1. Mix up pork chops and blended spinach.
2. Then preheat the grill to 400F.
3. Put the meat cubes in the grill and roast them for 6 minutes per side or until the meat is light brown.

per serving: 256 calories, 18g protein, 0g carbohydrates, 19.9g fat, 0g fiber, 69mg cholesterol, 57mg sodium, 279mg potassium.

Cranberry Pork

Yield: 4 servings | **Prep time:** 10 minutes | **Cook time:** 30 minutes

- 1-pound pork loin, chopped
- 1/3 cup cranberries
- 1 tablespoon margarine
- 1 teaspoon potato starch
- 1 teaspoon dried rosemary
- 1 teaspoon ground black pepper

1. Sprinkle the chopped meat with dried rosemary and ground black pepper and transfer in the skillet.
2. Add margarine and roast the meat for 15 minutes. Stir it from time to time.
3. Meanwhile, blend the cranberries and mix them up with starch. If the cranberries are not juicy, add water.
4. Bring the mixture to boil and pour it over the meat.
5. Simmer the meat for 5 minutes on low heat.

per serving: 312 calories, 31.3g protein, 2.6g carbohydrates, 18.7g fat, 0.6g fiber, 91mg cholesterol, 104mg sodium, 506mg potassium.

Stuffed Tomatoes

Yield: 2 servings | **Prep time:** 20 minutes | **Cook time:** 35 minutes
- 4 oz lean ground beef
- 2 tablespoons low-fat yogurt
- 1 teaspoon dried thyme
- ½ teaspoon chili powder
- 2 tomatoes
- ¼ cup of water

1. Cut the tops of tomatoes and scoop the tomato meat from them
2. Then mix up lean ground beef, thyme, and chili powder.
3. Fill the prepared tomatoes with meat mixture.
4. Then top them with yogurt and put in the casserole mold.
5. Add water and cover them with foil.
6. Bake the tomatoes for 35 minutes at 375F.

per serving: 142 calories, 19.3g protein, 6.5g carbohydrates, 4.1g fat, 1.9g fiber, 52mg cholesterol, 62mg sodium, 573mg potassium.

Chinese Style Beef

Yield: 2 servings | **Prep time:** 10 minutes | **Cook time:** 30 minutes
- 1 tablespoon scallions, chopped
- 1 oz fresh ginger, diced
- 1 onion, sliced
- ½ cup low-sodium chicken broth
- 8 oz beef tenderloin, sliced
- 1 teaspoon ground black pepper
- 3 tablespoons lemon juice
- Cooking spray

1. Spray the skillet with cooking spray and put sliced beef inside.
2. Sprinkle it with ground black pepper, lemon juice, and ginger.
3. Roast the meat for 10 minutes. Stir it from time to time.
4. After this, add onion, broth, and honey. Stir the mixture well.
5. Close the lid and cook it for 20 minutes on medium-low heat.
6. Top the cooked meat with scallions.

per serving: 318 calories, 35.6g protein, 16.8g carbohydrates, 11.5g fat, 34.g fiber, 104mg cholesterol, 97mg sodium, 725mg potassium.

Thai Steak

Yield: 3 servings | **Prep time:** 15 minutes | **Cook time:** 20 minutes
- 1 teaspoon minced ginger
- 1 teaspoon ground coriander
- 2 tablespoons olive oil
- 1 tablespoon liquid honey
- 3 tablespoons lemon juice
- 1 teaspoon chives, chopped
- 3 pork loin steaks

1. Mix up ground coriander, olive oil, minced ginger, liquid honey, lemon juice, and chives in the bowl.
2. Then coat the pork loin steaks in the oil mixture and leave for 10 minutes to marinate.
3. Preheat the grill to 400F.
4. Put the marinated steaks in the grill and cook them for 9 minutes per side.

per serving: 327 calories, 21.6g protein, 6.5g carbohydrates, 23.6g fat, 0.2g fiber, 81mg cholesterol, 62mg sodium, 309mg potassium.

Stuffed Pork Loin with Nuts

Yield: 6 servings | **Prep time:** 20 minutes | **Cook time:** 60 minutes
- 1-pound pork loin
- 1 oz nuts, chopped
- 1 oz walnuts, chopped
- 1 tablespoon low-fat yogurt
- 1 teaspoon minced ginger
- 1 tablespoon olive oil
- 1 teaspoon ground paprika
- ½ teaspoon ground black pepper

1. Beat the pork loin well and rub with minced ginger, ground paprika, and ground black pepper.
2. Then sprinkle the meat with nuts and walnuts and roll up into the roll.
3. Secure the meat roll with the help of the toothpicks if needed and brush with yogurt and olive oil.
4. Wrap the meat roll in the foil and bake in the preheated to 385F oven for 60 minutes.

per serving: 264 calories, 22.9g protein, 2.4g carbohydrates, 18.2g fat, 1g fiber, 61mg cholesterol, 81mg sodium, 393mg potassium.

Marinated Beef Steak Strips

Yield: 3 servings | **Prep time:** 35 minutes | **Cook time:** 16 minutes
- 14 oz beef flank steak
- 2 garlic cloves, diced
- 1 teaspoon chili pepper
- 3 tablespoons balsamic vinegar
- 2 tablespoons avocado oil
- 1 tablespoon liquid honey
- 1 tablespoon tomato puree

1. Make the marinade: mix up garlic, chili pepper, balsamic vinegar, avocado oil, liquid honey, and tomato puree.
2. Put the beef in the marinade and leave for 30 minutes to marinate.
3. Meanwhile, heat up the grill to 400F.
4. Put the marinated steaks in the grill and roast for 8 minutes per side.
5. Slice the cooked beef steaks into the strips.

per serving: 288 calories, 40.5g protein, 7.7g carbohydrates, 9.5g fat, 0.6g fiber, 118mg cholesterol, 91mg sodium, 613mg potassium.

Fennel Pork Chops

Yield: 4 servings | **Prep time:** 10 minutes | **Cook time:** 35 minutes
- 4 top pork loin chops
- 1 tablespoon fennel seeds
- 1 tablespoon margarine
- ½ cup water, hot

1. Toss margarine in the skillet and add fennel seeds.
2. Roast the condiments for 2 minutes or until they start to smell.
3. After this, add pork chops and broil them on high heat for 4 minutes per side.
4. Add hot water and bring the meat to boil.
5. Transfer the skillet with pork chops in the preheated to 375F oven and cook it for 25 minutes.

per serving: 224 calories, 26.2g protein, 0.8g carbohydrates, 12g fat, 0.6g fiber, 65mg cholesterol, 84mg sodium, 451mg potassium.

Curries Pork

Yield: 4 servings | **Prep time:** 10 minutes | **Cook time:** 25 minutes
- 12 oz pork loin, chopped
- 1 teaspoon curry paste
- ½ teaspoon minced ginger
- 1 tablespoon olive oil
- 1 cup tomatoes, chopped
- ¼ cup of water

1. Heat up olive oil in the saucepan.
2. Add chopped meat and roast it for 5 minutes. Stir it occasionally.
3. After this, add minced ginger and chopped tomatoes. Mix up the mixture and cook it for 5 minutes more.
4. Then add water and curry paste. Stir the ingredients with the help of the spatula until homogenous and close the lid.
5. Saute the meat for 15 minutes on medium heat.

per serving: 253 calories, 23.7g protein, 2.3g carbohydrates, 16.2g fat, 0.6g fiber, 68mg cholesterol, 55mg sodium, 470mg potassium.

Caribbean Pork Chops

Yield: 2 servings | **Prep time:** 10 minutes | **Cook time:** 25 minutes
- 2 pork loin chops
- 1 tablespoon Caribbean seasonings
- 1 tablespoon olive oil

1. Rub the pork chops with seasonings.
2. Heat up the olive oil in the skillet for 2 minutes.
3. Then add pork chops and cook them for 5 minutes per side.
4. After this, transfer the skillet with meat in the preheated to 375F oven and bake it for 15 minutes.

per serving: 329 calories, 18g protein, 3g carbohydrates, 26.9g fat, 0g fiber, 69mg cholesterol, 271mg sodium, 275mg potassium.

Bistro Beef Tenderloins

Yield: 2 servings | **Prep time:** 10 minutes | **Cook time:** 30 minutes
- 8 oz beef tenderloin
- 1 tablespoon avocado oil
- 1 teaspoon ground black pepper
- 2 tablespoons chives, chopped

1. Rub the meat with ground black pepper and brush with avocado oil.
2. Bake the meat at 365F for 30 minutes or until the meat will be tender.
3. Slice the cooked meat and top with chives.

per serving: 246 calories, 33.1g protein, 1.2g carbohydrates, 11.3g fat, 0.7g fiber, 104mg cholesterol, 68mg sodium, 449mg potassium.

Seasoned Baked Veal

Yield: 2 servings | **Prep time:** 10 minutes | **Cook time:** 30 minutes
- 1 oz veal, chopped
- 1 tablespoon Italian seasonings
- 1 teaspoon margarine, melted
- ¼ cup apple juice
- 1 onion, sliced

1. Mix up all ingredients and transfer them in the baking tray.
2. Cover the tray with foil and put in the preheated to 375F oven.
3. Bake the veal for 30 minutes.

per serving: 99 calories, 4.1g protein, 9.4g carbohydrates, 5.2g fat, 1.2g fiber, 20mg cholesterol, 40mg sodium, 164mg potassium.

Balsamic Vinegar Steak

Yield: 2 servings | **Prep time:** 20 minutes | **Cook time:** 20 minutes
- 2 beef sirloin steaks
- 1/3 cup balsamic vinegar
- 1 teaspoon dried thyme
- 1 tablespoon canola oil

1. Mix up balsamic vinegar and dried thyme.
2. Put the meat in the vinegar mixture and leave it to marinate for 15 minutes.
3. Then preheat the canola oil in the skillet.
4. Add steaks and cook them for 10 minutes per side on the medium heat.
5. Slice the cooked beef steaks.

per serving: 230 calories, 25.9g protein, 0.7g carbohydrates, 12.3g fat, 0.2g fiber, 76mg cholesterol, 58mg sodium, 376mg potassium.

Black Currant Beef Loin

Yield: 4 servings | **Prep time:** 15 minutes | **Cook time:** 50 minutes
- ½ cup black currant
- 1-pound beef loin
- 1 teaspoon beef seasonings
- 2 tablespoons olive oil
- ¼ cup of water
- 1 teaspoon potato starch
- 1 teaspoon chili powder

1. Rub the beef loin with beef seasonings and brush with olive oil.
2. Then put the meat in the tray and transfer in the preheated to 375F oven.
3. Bake the meat for 50 minutes.
4. Meanwhile, make the sauce: blend the black currant until smooth and transfer in the saucepan.
5. Add water and chili powder.
6. Bring the mixture to boil, add potato starch and whisk it well.
7. Simmer the currant mixture until thicken.
8. When the meat is cooked, slice it and sprinkle with hot currant sauce.

per serving: 292 calories, 30.4g protein, 6g carbohydrates, 16.6g fat, 0.2g fiber, 81mg cholesterol, 199mg sodium, 413mg potassium.

Fish and Seafood

Limes and Shrimps Skewers

Yield: 4 servings | **Prep time:** 15 minutes | **Cook time:** 6 minutes
- 1-pound shrimps, peeled
- 1 lime
- 1 teaspoon lemon juice
- ½ teaspoon white pepper

1. Cut the lime into wedges.
2. Then sprinkle the shrimps with lemon juice and white pepper.
3. String the lime and lime wedges in the wooden skewers one-by-one.
4. Preheat the grill to 400F.
5. Put the shrimp skewers in grill and cook for 3 minutes from each side or until the shrimps become light pink.

per serving: 141 calories, 26g protein, 3.7g carbohydrates, 2g fat, 0.6g fiber, 239mg cholesterol, 277mg sodium, 214mg potassium.

Crusted Salmon with Horseradish

Yield: 2 servings | **Prep time:** 10 minutes | **Cook time:** 13 minutes
- 8 oz salmon fillet
- 1 oz horseradish, grated
- ¼ teaspoon ground coriander
- 1 teaspoon coconut flakes
- 1 tablespoon olive oil

1. Mix up horseradish, ground coriander, and coconut flakes.
2. Then cut the salmon fillet on 2 servings.
3. Heat up olive oil in the skillet.
4. Put the salmon fillets in the skillet and top with the horseradish mixture.
5. Cook the fish for 5 minutes on the medium heat.
6. Then flip it on another side and cook for 8 minutes more.

per serving: 220 calories, 22.2g protein, 1.7g carbohydrates, 14.4g fat, 0.5g fiber, 50mg cholesterol, 95mg sodium, 473mg potassium.

Cucumber and Seafood Bowl

Yield: 3 servings | **Prep time:** 10 minutes | **Cook time:** 15 minutes
- 2 cucumbers, chopped
- 1 teaspoon mustard
- ½ teaspoon ground coriander
- 1 teaspoon margarine
- 6 oz shrimps, peeled
- 4 oz salmon, chopped
- 1 tablespoon low-fat yogurt

1. Heat up margarine in the skillet. Add chopped salmon and cook it for 2 minutes from each side.
2. Then add shrimps and sprinkle the seafood with ground coriander. Close the lid and cook the ingredients for 10 minutes on low heat.
3. Then transfer them in the serving bowls. Add cucumbers.
4. Mix up yogurt and mustard.
5. Sprinkle the meal with mustard mixture.

per serving: 168 calories, 22.1g protein, 8.9g carbohydrates, 5.2g fat, 1.2g fiber, 136mg cholesterol, 178mg sodium, 557mg potassium.

Fish Tacos

Yield: 4 servings | **Prep time:** 10 minutes | **Cook time:** 10 minutes
- 4 corn tortillas
- 1 cup white cabbage, shredded
- ¼ cup low-fat yogurt
- 1 teaspoon taco seasonings
- 1-pound cod fillet, chopped
- 1 tablespoon coconut oil

1. Sprinkle the chopped cod with taco seasonings.
2. Melt the coconut oil in the skillet.
3. Add cod and cook it for 5 minutes from each side or until the fish is light brown.
4. Then place the cooked fish on the corn tortillas.
5. Add shredded cabbage.
6. Sprinkle the ingredients with low-fat yogurt and wrap in the shape of tacos.

per serving: 212 calories, 27.5g protein, 13.3g carbohydrates, 5.5g fat, 2g fiber, 70mg cholesterol, 165mg sodium, 110mg potassium.

Tuna and Pineapple Kebob

Yield: 4 servings | **Prep time:** 10 minutes | **Cook time:** 8 minutes
- 12 oz tuna fillet

- 8 oz pineapple, peeled
- 1 teaspoon olive oil
- ¼ teaspoon ground fennel

1. Chop the tuna and pineapple on medium size cubes and sprinkle with olive oil and ground fennel.
2. Then string them in the skewers and place them in the preheated to 400F grill.
3. Cook the kebobs for 4 minutes per side.

per serving: 347 calories, 18.2g protein, 7.5g carbohydrates, 27.6g fat, 0.8g fiber, 0mg cholesterol, 1mg sodium, 64mg potassium.

Paprika Tilapia

Yield: 2 servings | **Prep time:** 7 minutes | **Cook time:** 10 minutes
- 2 tilapia fillets
- 1 teaspoon ground paprika
- ½ teaspoon chili powder
- 2 tablespoons avocado oil

1. Sprinkle the tilapia fillets with ground paprika and chili powder.
2. Then heat up avocado oil in the skillet for 2 minutes.
3. Put the fish fillets in the hot oil and cook for 3 minutes per side.

per serving: 1170 calories, 21.4g protein, 1.7g carbohydrates, 3.1g fat, 1.2g fiber, 55mg cholesterol, 47mg sodium, 81mg potassium.

Herbed Sole

Yield: 3 servings | **Prep time:** 10 minutes | **Cook time:** 10 minutes
- 10 oz sole fillet
- 2 tablespoons margarine
- 1 tablespoon dill weed
- 1 teaspoon garlic powder
- ½ teaspoon cumin seeds

1. Toss the margarine in the skillet.
2. Add cumin seeds and dill weed.
3. Melt the mixture and simmer it for 30 seconds.
4. Then cut the sole fillet on 2 servings and sprinkle with garlic powder.
5. Put the fish fillets in the melted margarine mixture.
6. Cook the fish for 3 minutes per side.

per serving: 185 calories, 23.3g protein, 1.5g carbohydrates, 9.2g fat, 0.3g fiber, 64mg cholesterol, 191mg sodium, 380mg potassium.

Rosemary Salmon

Yield: 4 servings | **Prep time:** 10 minutes | **Cook time:** 12 minutes
- 1-pound salmon fillet
- 4 teaspoons olive oil
- 4 teaspoons lemon juice
- 1 tablespoon dried rosemary

1. Cut the salmon fillet into 4 servings.
2. Then rub the fillets with olive oil, lemon juice, and dried rosemary.
3. Put the salmon on the tray and bake it for 12 minutes at 400F.

per serving: 194 calories, 22.1g protein, 0.6g carbohydrates, 11.8g fat, 0.4g fiber, 50mg cholesterol, 51mg sodium, 450mg potassium.

Tuna Stuffed Zucchini Boats

Yield: 2 servings | **Prep time:** 15 minutes | **Cook time:** 20 minutes
- 1 zucchini, trimmed
- 6 oz tuna, canned
- 2 oz low-fat cheese, shredded
- 1 teaspoon chili flakes
- 1 teaspoon olive oil

1. Cut the zucchini into halves and scoop the zucchini meat from them to get the zucchini boats.
2. Fill the zucchini boats with tuna and shredded cheese.
3. Sprinkle the zucchini with olive oil and transfer in the oven.
4. Cook the meal at 385F for 20 minutes.

per serving: 308 calories, 30.8g protein, 3.7g carbohydrates, 18.8g fat, 1.1g fiber, 56mg cholesterol, 229mg sodium, 570mg potassium.

Baked Cod

Yield: 2 servings | **Prep time:** 10 minutes | **Cook time:** 30 minutes
- 10 oz cod fillet
- 1 teaspoon Italian seasonings
- 1 tablespoon margarine

1. Rub the baking pan with margarine.
2. Then chop the cod and sprinkle with Italian seasonings.
3. Put the fish in the baking pan and cover with foil.
4. Bake the meal at 375F for 30 minutes.

per serving: 170 calories, 25.1g protein, 0.3g carbohydrates, 7.6g fat, 0g fiber, 70mg cholesterol, 155mg sodium, 4mg potassium.

Basil Halibut

Yield: 4 servings | **Prep time:** 10 minutes | **Cook time:** 10 minutes
- 1-pound halibut, chopped
- 1 tablespoon dried basil
- 1 teaspoon garlic powder
- 2 tablespoons olive oil

1. Pour olive oil in the skillet and heat it up.
2. Meanwhile, mix up halibut, dried basil, and garlic powder.
3. Toss the fish in the hot oil and coot it for 3 minutes per side.

per serving: 347 calories, 22.1g protein, 0.5g carbohydrates, 28.2g fat, 0.1g fiber, 70mg cholesterol, 123mg sodium, 420mg potassium.

Tilapia Veracruz

Yield: 4 servings | **Prep time:** 10 minutes | **Cook time:** 20 minutes
- 1 cup tomatoes, chopped
- 1 teaspoon dried oregano
- 1 onion, diced
- ½ cup bell pepper, chopped
- ¼ cup of water
- 1 tablespoon olive oil
- 4 tilapia fillets

1. Heat up olive oil in the skillet and add tilapia fillets.
2. Roast the fish for 4 minutes per side. Remove the fish from the skillet.
3. Add the onion in the skillet and cook it for 2 minutes.
4. Then add bell peppers, oregano, and tomatoes. Stir the ingredients well and cook them for 5 minutes.
5. After this, add water and fish.
6. Close the lid and cook the meal for 5 minutes more.

per serving: 148 calories, 21.9g protein, 5.7g carbohydrates, 4.7g fat, 1.5g fiber, 55mg cholesterol, 44mg sodium, 181mg potassium.

Lemon Swordfish

Yield: 4 servings | **Prep time:** 10 minutes | **Cook time:** 25 minutes
- 18 oz swordfish fillets
- 1 tablespoon margarine
- 1 teaspoon lemon zest
- 3 tablespoons lemon juice
- 1 teaspoon ground black pepper
- 2 tablespoons olive oil
- ½ teaspoon minced garlic

1. Cut the fish into 4 servings.
2. After this, in the mixing bowl, mix up lemon zest, lemon juice, ground black pepper, and olive oil. Add minced garlic.
3. Rub the fish fillets with lemon mixture.
4. Grease the baking pan with margarine and arrange the swordfish fillets.
5. Bake the fish for 25 minutes at 390F.

per serving: 288 calories, 32.6g protein, 0.8g carbohydrates, 16.5g fat, 0.2g fiber, 64mg cholesterol, 183mg sodium, 496mg potassium.

Spiced Scallops

Yield: 4 servings | **Prep time:** 10 minutes | **Cook time:** 5 minutes
- 1-pound scallops
- 1 teaspoon Cajun seasonings
- 1 tablespoon olive oil

1. Rub the scallops with Cajun seasonings.
2. Heat up olive oil in the skillet.
3. Add scallops and cook them for 2 minutes per each side.

per serving: 130 calories, 19g protein, 2.7g carbohydrates, 4.4g fat, 0g fiber, 37mg cholesterol, 195mg sodium, 365mg potassium.

Shrimp Putanesca

Yield: 3 servings | **Prep time:** 5 minutes | **Cook time:** 20 minutes
- 5 oz shrimps, peeled
- 1 teaspoon chili flakes
- ½ onion, diced
- 1 tablespoon coconut oil
- 1 teaspoon garlic, diced
- 1 cup tomatoes, chopped
- ¼ cup olives, sliced
- ¼ cup of water

1. Heat up coconut oil in the saucepan.
2. Add shrimps and chili flakes. Cook the shrimps for 4 minutes.
3. Stir them well and add diced onion, garlic, tomatoes, olives, and water.

4. Close the lid and sauté the meal for 15 minutes.
per serving: 128 calories, 11.7g protein, 5.8g carbohydrates, 6.7g fat, 1.5g fiber, 100mg cholesterol, 217mg sodium, 255mg potassium.

Curry Snapper

Yield: 4 servings | **Prep time:** 10 minutes | **Cook time:** 15 minutes
- 1-pound snapper fillet, chopped
- 1 teaspoon curry powder
- 1 cup celery stalk, chopped
- ½ cup low-fat yogurt
- ¼ cup of water
- 1 tablespoon olive oil

1. Roast the snapper fillet in the olive oil for 2 minutes per side.
2. Then add celery stalk, curry powder, low-fat yogurt, and water.
3. Stir the fish until you get the homogenous texture.
4. Close the lid and simmer the fish for 10 minutes on medium heat.

per serving: 195 calories, 29.5g protein, 3.2g carbohydrates, 5.9g fat, 0.6g fiber, 52mg cholesterol, 105mg sodium, 145mg potassium.

Grouper with Tomato Sauce

Yield: 2 servings | **Prep time:** 10 minutes | **Cook time:** 15 minutes
- 12 oz grouper, chopped
- 2 cups grape tomatoes, chopped
- 1 chili pepper, chopped
- 1 tablespoon margarine
- 1 teaspoon ground coriander

1. Toss the margarine in the saucepan.
2. Add chopped grouper and sprinkle it with ground coriander.
3. Roast the fish for 2 minutes per side.
4. Then add grape tomatoes and chili pepper.
5. Stir the ingredients well and close the lid.
6. Cook the meal for 10 minutes on low heat.

per serving: 285 calories, 43.9g protein, 7.2g carbohydrates, 8.3g fat, 2.2g fiber, 80mg cholesterol, 166mg sodium, 1243mg potassium.

Braised Seabass

Yield: 2 servings | **Prep time:** 8 minutes | **Cook time:** 28 minutes
- 10 oz seabass fillet
- 1 cup tomatoes, chopped
- 1 yellow onion, sliced
- 1 tablespoon avocado oil
- 1 teaspoon ground black pepper

1. Heat up olive oil in the skillet.
2. Add seabass fillet and roast it for 4 minutes per side.
3. Then remove the fish from the skillet and add sliced onion.
4. Cook it for 2 minutes.
5. After this, add tomatoes, and ground black pepper.
6. Bring the mixture to boil.
7. Add cooked seabass and close the lid.
8. Cook the meal for 15 minutes.

per serving: 285 calories, 27.7g protein, 9.7g carbohydrates, 15.3g fat, 3.8g fiber, 0mg cholesterol, 8mg sodium, 329mg potassium.

Five-Spices Sole

Yield: 3 servings | **Prep time:** 10 minutes | **Cook time:** 11 minutes
- 3 sole fillets
- 1 tablespoon five-spice seasonings
- 1 tablespoon coconut oil

1. Rub the sole fillets with seasonings.
2. Then heat up the coconut oil in the skillet for 2 minutes.
3. Place the sole fillets in the hot oil and cook them for 4.5 minutes per side.

per serving: 204 calories, 31.8g protein, 1g carbohydrates, 6.5g fat, 2.2g fiber, 86mg cholesterol, 133mg sodium, 437mg potassium.

Clams Stew

Yield: 5 servings | **Prep time:** 8 minutes | **Cook time:** 10 minutes
- 1-pound clams
- 1 teaspoon dried thyme
- 1 teaspoon ground paprika
- ½ cup light cream (low-fat)
- 1 tablespoon lemon juice

1. Put dried thyme, ground paprika, and cream.
2. Bring the liquid to boil.

3.	Then add lemon juice and whisk the mixture well.
4.	Add clams and close the lid.
5.	Simmer the clams stew for 5 minutes.
per serving: 94 calories, 0.6g protein, 12g carbohydrates, 5.1g fat, 0.6g fiber, 16mg cholesterol, 345mg sodium, 96mg potassium

Salmon in Capers

Yield: 4 servings | **Prep time:** 10 minutes | **Cook time:** 15 minutes
- *2 tablespoons avocado oil*
- *1-pound salmon fillet, chopped*
- *1 tablespoon capers, drained*
- *½ cup low-fat milk*

1.	Heat up a pan with the oil over medium-high heat, add salmon and roast it for 5 minutes.
2.	Add capers and milk and saute the meal for 10 minutes over the medium heat.
per serving: 173 calories, 23.2g protein, 2g carbohydrates, 8.2g fat, 0.4g fiber, 52mg cholesterol, 127mg sodium, 504mg potassium

Horseradish Cod

Yield: 4 servings | **Prep time:** 10 minutes | **Cook time:** 10 minutes
- *1 tablespoon avocado oil*
- *12 oz cod fillet*
- *½ cup low-fat cream cheese*
- *¼ teaspoon ground black pepper*
- *2 tablespoons dill, chopped*
- *1 tablespoon horseradish*

1.	Heat up a pan with the oil over medium-high heat, add cod, season with black pepper and cook for 5 minutes on each side.
2.	In a bowl, combine the cream cheese with the dill and horseradish.
3.	Top the cooked cod with horseradish mixture.
per serving: 180 calories, 17.8g protein, 2.3g carbohydrates, 11.4g fat, 0.5g fiber, 74mg cholesterol, 154mg sodium, 108mg potassium

Salmon and Corn Salad

Yield: 4 servings | **Prep time:** 10 minutes | **Cook time:** 0 minutes
- *2 tablespoons canola oil*
- *½ teaspoon lemon juice*
- *1 cup corn kernels, cooked*
- *1-pound salmon, canned, shredded*
- *1 tablespoon scallions, chopped*

1.	Put all ingredients in the bowl and mix up the salad.
per serving: 246 calories, 23.3g protein, 7.4g carbohydrates, 14.5g fat, 1.1g fiber, 50mg cholesterol, 56mg sodium, 544mg potassium

Mustard Tuna Salad

Yield: 2 servings | **Prep time:** 10 minutes | **Cook time:** 0 minutes
- *½ teaspoon lemon juice*
- *1 tablespoon mustard*
- *¼ teaspoon cayenne pepper*
- *¼ cup chickpeas, cooked*
- *5 ounces white tuna canned in water, drained*
- *1 teaspoon olive oil*

1.	Mix up olive oil, mustard, and lemon juice in the shallow bowl.
2.	Mix up all remaining ingredients in the salad bowl and top with mustard mixture. Shake the salad well.
per serving: 229 calories, 23g protein, 17.3g carbohydrates, 7.6g fat, 5.2g fiber, 30mg cholesterol, 274mg sodium, 431mg potassium

Shallot Tuna

Yield: 4 servings | **Prep time:** 10 minutes | **Cook time:** 10 minutes
- *1-pound tuna fillet, chopped*
- *1 tablespoon olive oil*
- *½ cup shallot, chopped*
- *2 tablespoons lime juice*
- *½ cup of water*

1.	Heat up a pan with the oil over medium-high heat, add shallots and sauté for 3 minutes.
2.	Add the fish and cook it for 4 minutes on each side.
3.	Then sprinkle the fish with lime juice and water.
4.	Close the lid and simmer the tuna for 3 minutes.
per serving: 458 calories, 24.3g protein, 3.9g carbohydrates, 38.7g fat, 0g fiber, 0mg cholesterol, 5mg sodium, 73mg potassium

Cod Relish

Yield: 4 servings | **Prep time:** 10 minutes | **Cook time:** 5 minutes
- 1 teaspoon dried oregano
- 1 cup green peas, cooked
- 1 onion, diced
- 3 tablespoons olive oil
- ½ teaspoon white pepper
- 1-pound cod fillet, chopped

1. Heat up a pan with 1 tablespoon oil over medium-high heat, add the cod fillets, cook it for 2 minutes on each side.
2. After this, put the fish in the serving plates.
3. In the mixing bowl, mix up all remaining ingredients and shale well.
4. Top the fish with onion mixture.

per serving: 223 calories, 22.6g protein, 8.2g carbohydrates, 11.7g fat, 2.7g fiber, 56mg cholesterol, 74mg sodium, 138mg potassium

Mint Cod

Yield: 4 servings | **Prep time:** 10 minutes | **Cook time:** 7 minutes
- 1 tablespoon avocado oil
- 1 tablespoon lemon juice
- 1 tablespoon mint, chopped
- 1-pound cod fillet
- 2 tablespoons water

1. Heat up a pan with the oil over medium heat, add mint and cod.
2. Cook the fish for 3 minutes per side.
3. Then add water and lemon juice. Cook the cod for 2 minutes more.

per serving: 97 calories, 20.4g protein, 0.4g carbohydrates, 1.5g fat, 0.3g fiber, 56mg cholesterol, 72mg sodium, 22mg potassium

Dill Steamed Salmon

Yield: 4 servings | **Prep time:** 10 minutes | **Cook time:** 0 minutes
- 2 tablespoons dill, chopped
- 1 tablespoon low-fat cream cheese
- 1 teaspoon chili flakes
- 1 pound steamed salmon, chopped
- 1 red onion, diced

1. Mix up all ingredients in the bowl and carefully stir until homogenous.

per serving: 174 calories, 22.8g protein, 3.5g carbohydrates, 8g fat, 0.8g fiber, 53mg cholesterol, 62mg sodium, 531mg potassium

Cod in Tomatoes

Yield: 4 servings | **Prep time:** 10 minutes | **Cook time:** 16 minutes
- 2 tablespoons avocado oil
- ½ teaspoon minced garlic
- ½ cup of water
- 4 cod fillets, boneless
- 1 cup plum tomatoes, chopped
- 1 teaspoon scallions, chopped

1. Heat up a pan with the oil over medium-high heat, add the garlic and the fish and cook for 3 minutes per side.
2. Then top the fish with the remaining ingredients and cook for 10 minutes more.

per serving: 110 calories, 20.7g protein, 2.9g carbohydrates, 2g fat, 0.8g fiber, 40mg cholesterol, 87mg sodium, 117mg potassium

Spinach Halibut

Yield: 4 servings | **Prep time:** 10 minutes | **Cook time:** 6 minutes
- 4 halibut fillets
- 2 tablespoons spinach, blended
- 1 teaspoon margarine

1. Melt the margarine in the skillet and add fish fillets.
2. Cook them for 3 minutes per side.
3. Top the cooked halibut with spinach.

per serving: 327 calories, 60.5g protein, 0g carbohydrates, 7.7g fat, 0g fiber, 93mg cholesterol, 168mg sodium, 1312mg potassium

Paprika Tuna Steaks

Yield: 4 servings | **Prep time:** 10 minutes | **Cook time:** 4 minutes
- 1 teaspoon avocado oil
- 4 tuna steaks, boneless
- 1 teaspoon ground paprika

1. Rub the fish with paprika and sprinkle with avocado oil.
2. Then transfer the tuna steaks in the preheated to 400F grill and cook for 2 minutes per side.

per serving: 159 calories, 25.5g protein, 0.4g carbohydrates, 5.6g fat, 0.3g fiber, 42mg cholesterol, 43mg sodium, 291mg potassium

Grilled Tilapia

Yield: 4 servings | **Prep time:** 10 minutes | **Cook time:** 6 minutes

- *1 tablespoon sesame oil*
- *½ teaspoon ground black pepper*
- *½ teaspoon garlic powder*
- *4 medium tilapia fillets*

1. Sprinkle the fish with garlic powder, ground black pepper, and sesame oil.
2. Grill it for 3 minutes per side in the preheated to 400F grill.

per serving: 125 calories,21.1g protein, 0.4g carbohydrates, 4.4g fat, 0.1g fiber, 55mg cholesterol, 40mg sodium, 7mg potassium

Cod in Orange Juice

Yield: 4 servings | **Prep time:** 5 minutes | **Cook time:** 12 minutes

- *4 cod fillets, boneless*
- *1 cup of orange juice*
- *1 tablespoon chives, chopped*
- *1 tablespoon olive oil*
- *½ teaspoon white pepper*

1. Heat up a pan with the oil over medium heat.
2. Sprinkle the fish with white pepper and out in the hot oil.
3. Add orange juice and chives.
4. Cook the fish for 10 minutes.

per serving: 149 calories,20.5g protein, 6.7g carbohydrates, 4.7g fat, 0.2g fiber, 40mg cholesterol, 81mg sodium, 129mg potassium

Tomato Halibut Fillets

Yield: 4 servings | **Prep time:** 10 minutes | **Cook time:** 10 minutes

- *2 teaspoon sesame oil*
- *4 halibut fillets, skinless*
- *1 cup cherry tomatoes, halved*
- *1 teaspoon dried basil*

1. Sprinkle the fish with basil and put in the hot skillet.
2. Add sesame oil and cherry tomatoes.
3. Roast the meal for 4 minutes and then stir well and cook for 5 minutes more.

per serving: 346 calories,60.9g protein, 1.8g carbohydrates, 9.1g fat, 0.5g fiber, 93mg cholesterol, 158mg sodium, 1414mg potassium

Salmon with Basil and Garlic

Yield: 4 servings | **Prep time:** 5 minutes | **Cook time:** 14 minutes

- *2 tablespoons avocado oil*
- *4 salmon fillets, skinless*
- *1 teaspoon dried basil*
- *½ teaspoon garlic powder*

1. Heat up a pan with the olive oil, add the fish and cook for 4 minutes per side.
2. Sprinkle the cooked salmon with garlic powder and basil.

per serving: 246 calories,34.7g protein, 0.7g carbohydrates, 11.9g fat, 0.3g fiber, 78mg cholesterol, 79mg sodium, 710mg potassium

Mustard Arctic Char

Yield: 2 servings | **Prep time:** 10 minutes | **Cook time:** 10 minutes

- *1 tablespoon mustard*
- *1 tablespoon olive oil*
- *¼ teaspoon dried rosemary*
- *2 arctic char fillets*

1. Sprinkle the fish with rosemary, olive oil, and mustard.
2. Then transfer the fish fillets in the baking pan and bake for 10 at 400F.

per serving: 291 calories,25.4g protein, 2.1g carbohydrates, 10.6g fat, 0.9g fiber, 8mg cholesterol, 22mg sodium, 40mg potassium

Cod in Yogurt Sauce

Yield: 4 servings | **Prep time:** 10 minutes | **Cook time:** 15 minutes

- *1 teaspoon sesame oil*
- *4 cod fillets, boneless and skinless*
- *½ onion, diced*
- *½ cup low-fat yogurt*
- *1 tablespoon dried cilantro*
- *½ teaspoon minced garlic*

1. Rub the cod fillets with dried cilantro, minced garlic, and sesame oil.
2. Put the fish in the skillet and cook it for 3 minutes per side.
3. Add onion and fat yogurt. Cook the meal for 12 minutes more.

per serving: 128 calories,21.9g protein, 3.6g carbohydrates, 2.5g fat, 0.3g fiber, 42mg cholesterol, 102mg sodium, 94mg potassium

Parsley Trout

Yield: 6 servings | **Prep time:** 10 minutes | **Cook time:** 10 minutes

- *1 tablespoon dried parsley*
- *6 trout fillets*
- *2 tablespoons margarine*

1. Rub the trout fillets with parsley.
2. Then toss the margarine in the skillet and melt it.
3. Add fish fillets and cook them for 4 minutes per side.

per serving: 152 calories,16.6g protein, 0.1g carbohydrates, 9g fat, 0g fiber, 46mg cholesterol, 86mg sodium, 293mg potassium

Halibut with Radish Slices

Yield: 4 servings | **Prep time:** 10 minutes | **Cook time:** 6 minutes

- 4 halibut fillets, boneless
- 1 cup radishes, sliced
- 1 tablespoon apple cider vinegar
- ¼ teaspoon ground coriander
- 1 tablespoon olive oil
- 1 teaspoon low-fat cream cheese

1. Sprinkle the fish fillets with apple cider vinegar, ground coriander, and olive oil.
2. Then grill the halibut in the preheated to 385F grill for 3 minutes per side.
3. Transfer the fish in the plates and top with sliced radish and cream cheese.

per serving: 356 calories,60.8g protein, 1g carbohydrates, 10.5g fat, 0.5g fiber, 94mg cholesterol, 170mg sodium, 1378mg potassium

Green Onion Salmon

Yield: 4 servings | **Prep time:** 10 minutes | **Cook time:** 10 minutes

- 4 green olives, pitted, sliced
- 2 oz green onions, blended
- ½ teaspoon chili flakes
- ¼ teaspoon ground black pepper
- 3 tablespoons avocado oil
- 4 salmon fillets, skinless and boneless
- 1 oz parsley, chopped

1. Blend together green onions, chili flakes, ground black pepper, avocado oil, and parsley.
2. Then rub the salmon fillets with green onion mixture and transfer in the preheated skillet.
3. Cook it for 4 minutes per side.
4. Top the cooked fish with sliced olives.

per serving: 272 calories,35.1g protein, 3.2g carbohydrates, 13.4g fat, 1.1g fiber, 78mg cholesterol, 375mg sodium, 797mg potassium

Broccoli and Cod Mash

Yield: 4 servings | **Prep time:** 10 minutes | **Cook time:** 20 minutes

- 2 cups broccoli, chopped
- 4 cod fillets, boneless, chopped
- 1 white onion, chopped
- 2 tablespoons olive oil
- 1 cup of water
- 1 tablespoon low-fat cream cheese
- ½ teaspoon ground black pepper

1. Roast the cod in the saucepan with olive oil for 1 minute per side.
2. Then add all remaining ingredients except cream cheese and boil the meal for 18 minutes.
3. After this, drain water, add cream cheese, and stir the meal well.

per serving: 186 calories,21.8g protein, 5.8g carbohydrates, 9.1g fat, 1.8g fiber, 43mg cholesterol, 105mg sodium, 191mg potassium

Greek Style Salmon

Yield: 4 servings | **Prep time:** 10 minutes | **Cook time:** 10 minutes

- 4 medium salmon fillets, skinless and boneless
- 1 tablespoon lemon juice
- 1 tablespoon dried oregano
- 1 teaspoon dried thyme
- ¼ teaspoon onion powder
- 1 tablespoon olive oil

1. Heat up olive oil in the skillet.
2. Sprinkle the salmon with dried oregano, thyme, onion powder, and lemon juice.
3. Put the fish in the skillet and cook for 4 minutes per side.

per serving: 271 calories,34.7g protein, 1.1g carbohydrates, 14.7g fat, 0.6g fiber, 78mg cholesterol, 80mg sodium, 711mg potassium

Spicy Ginger Seabass

Yield: 4 servings | **Prep time:** 5 minutes | **Cook time:** 10 minutes

- 1 tablespoon ginger, grated
- 2 tablespoons sesame oil
- ¼ teaspoon chili powder
- 4 sea bass fillets, boneless
- 1 tablespoon margarine

1. Heat up sesame oil and margarine in the skillet.
2. Add chili powder and ginger.
3. Then add seabass and cook the fish for 3 minutes per side.
4. Then close the lid and simmer the fish for 3 minutes over low heat.

per serving: 216 calories, 24g protein, 1.1g carbohydrates, 12.3g fat, 0.2g fiber, 54mg cholesterol, 123mg sodium, 354mg potassium

Yogurt Shrimps

Yield: 5 servings | **Prep time:** 5 minutes | **Cook time:** 10 minutes

- 1 pound shrimp, peeled
- 1 tablespoon margarine
- ¼ cup low-fat yogurt
- 1 teaspoon lemon zest, grated
- 1 chili pepper, chopped

1. Melt the margarine in the skillet, add chili pepper, and roast it for 1 minute.
2. Then add shrimps and lemon zest.
3. Roast the shrimps for 2 minutes per side.
4. After this, add yogurt, stir the shrimps well and cook for 5 minutes.

per serving: 137 calories, 21.4g protein, 2.4g carbohydrates, 4g fat, 0.1g fiber, 192mg cholesterol, 257mg sodium, 187mg potassium

Aromatic Salmon with Fennel Seeds

Yield: 5 servings | **Prep time:** 8 minutes | **Cook time:** 10 minutes

- 4 medium salmon fillets, skinless and boneless
- 1 tablespoon fennel seeds
- 2 tablespoons olive oil
- 1 tablespoon lemon juice
- 1 tablespoon water

1. Heat up olive oil in the skillet.
2. Add fennel seeds and roast them for 1 minute.
3. Add salmon fillets and sprinkle with lemon juice.
4. Add water and roast the fish for 4 minutes per side over the medium heat.

per serving: 301 calories, 4.8g protein, 0.8g carbohydrates, 18.2g fat, 0.6g fiber, 78mg cholesterol, 81mg sodium, 713mg potassium

Fish Spread

Yield: 8 servings | **Prep time:** 10 minutes | **Cook time:** 0 minutes

- 2-pounds trout, boiled
- 2 tablespoons low-fat cream cheese
- 1 tablespoon fresh dill, chopped
- 1 teaspoon minced garlic
- ¼ cup low-fat yogurt

1. Put all ingredients in the food processor and blend until smooth.
2. Transfer the fish spread in the bowl and flatten it well.
3. Refrigerate the spread for 5-10 minutes before serving.

per serving: 231 calories, 30.9g protein, 1g carbohydrates, 10.6g fat, 0.1g fiber, 87mg cholesterol, 90mg sodium, 560mg potassium

Allspice Shrimps

Yield: 4 servings | **Prep time:** 5 minutes | **Cook time:** 8 minutes

- 1 teaspoon allspice, ground
- 2 tablespoons olive oil
- 1-pound shrimps, peeled

1. Heat up olive oil in the skillet.
2. Mix up allspices and shrimps in the bowl.
3. Then transfer the seafood in the hot oil and cook for 3 minutes per side or until the shrimps are bright pink.

per serving: 196 calories, 25.9g protein, 2.1g carbohydrates, 9g fat, 0.1g fiber, 239mg cholesterol, 277mg sodium, 197mg potassium

Saffron Spiced Shrimps

Yield: 4 servings | **Prep time:** 10 minutes | **Cook time:** 15 minutes

- 1 teaspoon lemon juice
- 1 tablespoon sesame oil
- ½ teaspoon smoked paprika
- 1 yellow onion, chopped
- 1 pound shrimp, peeled and deveined
- 1 teaspoon saffron powder

1. Heat up sesame oil and add the onion. Roast it for 2-3 minutes over the medium heat.
2. Meanwhile, mix up saffron powder, shrimps, lemon juice, and smoked paprika.
3. Add the shrimps in the skillet and mix up well.

4. Cook the meal for 10 minutes over the medium heat.
per serving: 177 calories, 26.2g protein, 4.6g carbohydrates, 5.4g fat, 0.7g fiber, 239mg cholesterol, 278mg sodium, 243mg potassium

Lemon Zest Seabass

Yield: 4 servings | **Prep time:** 8 minutes | **Cook time:** 10 minutes
- 2 tablespoons olive oil
- 1-pounds sea bass fillets, skinless and boneless
- 1 tablespoon lemon zest, grated
- ¼ cup lemon juice
- 1 garlic clove, diced
- 1 teaspoon margarine

1. Melt the margarine in the skillet.
2. Add olive oil and garlic. Roast it for 1 minute.
3. Then sprinkle the seabass fillets with lemon zest and lemon juice and put in the skillet with garlic.
4. Roast the fish for 4 minutes per side over the medium heat.

per serving: 215 calories, 27g protein, 0.9g carbohydrates, 11g fat, 0.2g fiber, 60mg cholesterol, 113mg sodium, 399mg potassium

Spanish Style Mussels

Yield: 8 servings | **Prep time:** 10 minutes | **Cook time:** 20 minutes
- 3 tablespoons olive oil
- 2 pounds mussels, scrubbed
- ½ teaspoon ground black pepper
- 1 cup tomatoes, chopped
- 1 onion, diced
- 1 cup of water
- ½ cup fresh dill, chopped

1. Heat up a pan with the oil over medium-high heat, add onion, stir and cook for 3 minutes.
2. Add water, tomatoes, and black pepper, stir, bring to a simmer and cook for 10 minutes.
3. Add mussels and parsley, toss, cover the pan, cook for 7 minutes more.

per serving: 160 calories, 14.5g protein, 8.1g carbohydrates, 8g fat, 1g fiber, 32mg cholesterol, 333mg sodium, 537mg potassium

Salmon with Grated Beets

Yield: 5 servings | **Prep time:** 10 minutes | **Cook time:** 10 minutes
- 2 oz beetroot, grated
- ½ teaspoon minced garlic
- 1 teaspoon olive oil
- 1-pound salmon fillet
- 1 tablespoon mustard
- 1 tablespoon margarine

1. Rub the salmon with mustard and put it in the skillet.
2. Add margarine and roast the fish for 4 minutes per side.
3. Meanwhile, mix up minced garlic, grated beetroot, and olive oil.
4. Top the cooked salmon fillets with grated beetroot.

per serving: 164 calories, 18.4g protein, 2g carbohydrates, 9.5g fat, 0.6g fiber, 40mg cholesterol, 75mg sodium, 401mg potassium

Cold Crab Mix

Yield: 4 servings | **Prep time:** 15 minutes | **Cook time:** 0 minutes
- 2 cups tomatoes, chopped
- 3 cups watermelon, chopped
- 3 tablespoons apple cider vinegar
- 1 tablespoon sesame seeds
- 1 tablespoon avocado oil
- 1 cup crabmeat, chopped

1. Mix up all ingredients in the big bowl and shake well.
2. Refrigerate the meal for 10 minutes in the fridge.

per serving: 111 calories, 5.1g protein, 19.3g carbohydrates, 2.1g fat, 2.2g fiber, 9mg cholesterol, 364mg sodium, 408mg potassium

Onion Tilapia

Yield: 4 servings | **Prep time:** 10 minutes | **Cook time:** 10 minutes
- 4 tilapia fillets, boneless
- 1 tablespoon apple cider vinegar
- 1 tablespoon olive oil
- 1 teaspoon onion powder
- 1 white onion, sliced
- ½ teaspoon ground black pepper

1. Roast the onion with olive oil in the skillet for 2 minutes.
2. Meanwhile sprinkle the tilapia with apple cider vinegar, ground black pepper, and onion powder.
3. Add it in the onion and cook the meal for 4 minutes.
4. Then flip the fish fillets on another side and cook for 4 minutes more.

per serving: 138 calories, 21.4g protein, 3.3g carbohydrates, 4.6g fat, 0.7g fiber, 55mg cholesterol, 42mg sodium, 52mg potassium

Scallop Salad

Yield: 6 servings | **Prep time:** 10 minutes | **Cook time:** 13 minutes

- *12 ounces sea scallops*
- *4 tablespoons sesame oil*
- *4 teaspoons apple cider vinegar*
- *1 cup quinoa, cooked*
- *½ teaspoon garlic powder*
- *1 cup green peas, cooked*
- *1 tablespoon dried cilantro*

1. In a bowl, mix scallops apple cider vinegar and sesame oil.
2. Heat up a pan over medium heat, add scallops, stir and cook for 8 minutes (4 minutes per side).
3. Add all remaining ingredients, stir well. Cook the salad for 5 minutes over the low heat.

per serving: 255 calories, 14.9g protein, 23.2g carbohydrates, 11.3g fat, 3.2g fiber, 19mg cholesterol, 94mg sodium, 407mg potassium

Vinegar Trout

Yield: 4 servings | **Prep time:** 5 minutes | **Cook time:** 10 minutes

- *3 tablespoons apple cider vinegar*
- *2 tablespoons avocado oil*
- *4 trout fillets, boneless*
- *1 teaspoon ground coriander*

1. Heat up a pan with the oil over medium heat, add the trout, sprinkle it with apple cider vinegar, and ground coriander.
2. Cook the fish for 4 minutes on each side.

per serving: 129 calories, 16.6g protein, 0.5g carbohydrates, 6.1g fat, 0.3g fiber, 46mg cholesterol, 42mg sodium, 318mg potassium

Fish Salsa

Yield: 12 servings | **Prep time:** 10 minutes | **Cook time:** 0 minutes

- *1 cup tomatoes, chopped*
- *1-pound salmon, cooked, chopped*
- *½ cup tomatillos, chopped*
- *1 cup watermelon, seedless and chopped*
- *½ cup red onion, chopped*
- *1 cup mango, chopped*
- *¼ cup cilantro, chopped*
- *3 tablespoons lemon juice*
- *2 tablespoons avocado oil*

1. Put all ingredients in the bowl.
2. Stir the salsa well and leave it in a cool place for at least 5 minutes.

per serving: 67 calories, 7.2g protein, 4.2g carbohydrates, 2.6g fat, 0.7g fiber, 15mg cholesterol, 17mg sodium, 234mg potassium

Turmeric Pate

Yield: 6 servings | **Prep time:** 8 minutes | **Cook time:** 10 minutes

- *1-pound tuna, canned*
- *3 teaspoons lemon juice*
- *¼ cup low-fat yogurt*
- *1 teaspoon ground cinnamon*
- *½ teaspoon ground turmeric*

1. Put all ingredients in the food processor.
2. Blend the pate until smooth and transfer in the bowl.

per serving: 149 calories, 20.7g protein, 0.9g carbohydrates, 6.3g fat, 0.1g fiber, 24mg cholesterol, 46mg sodium, 283mg potassium

Celery Crab Salad

Yield: 4 servings | **Prep time:** 10 minutes | **Cook time:** 0 minutes

- *¼ teaspoon dried rosemary*
- *10 oz crab meat, cooked, chopped*
- *¼ teaspoon white pepper*
- *1 cup celery stalk, chopped*
- *¼ cup low-fat yogurt*

1. Mix up all ingredients in the salad bowl.
2. Refrigerate the salad for 5-10 minutes in the fridge before serving.

per serving: 79 calories, 9.9g protein, 3.2g carbohydrates, 1.5g fat, 0.5g fiber, 39mg

cholesterol, 474mg sodium, 104mg potassium

Lime Calamari

Yield: 4 servings | **Prep time:** 10 minutes | **Cook time:** 5 minutes

- *1 tablespoon lime juice*
- *1 teaspoon lime zest, grated*
- *1-pound calamari, sliced*
- *¼ teaspoon ground nutmeg*
- *1 tablespoon olive oil*
- *1 teaspoon dried mint*
- *¼ cup of water*

1. Mix up lime juice, lime zest, calamari, ground nutmeg, and olive oil in the bowl.
2. Add dried mint and water. Stir the mixture and transfer in the hot skillet.
3. Roast the calamari for 5 minutes over the medium heat. Stir the seafood from time to time.

per serving: 139 calories, 8.1g protein, 9g carbohydrates, 7.6g fat, 0.6g fiber, 0mg cholesterol, 256mg sodium, 7mg potassium

Juicy Scallops

Yield: 4 servings | **Prep time:** 10 minutes | **Cook time:** 5 minutes

- *12 oz sea scallops*
- *2 tablespoons olive oil*
- *½ teaspoon garlic powder*
- *¼ cup low-fat yogurt*

1. Sprinkle the scallops with garlic powder and olive oil and toss them in the hot skillet.
2. Roast the scallops for 3 minutes per side or until they are light brown.
3. Add yogurt and cook the seafood for 2 minutes more.

per serving: 147 calories, 15.2g protein, 3.3g carbohydrates, 7.8g fat, 0g fiber, 29mg cholesterol, 148mg sodium, 314mg potassium

Vegan and Vegetarian Main Dish

Mushroom Florentine

Yield: 4 servings | **Prep time:** 10 minutes | **Cook time:** 20 minutes
- 5 oz whole-grain pasta
- ¼ cup low-sodium vegetable broth
- 1 cup mushrooms, sliced
- ¼ cup of soy milk
- 1 teaspoon olive oil
- ½ teaspoon Italian seasonings

1. Cook the pasta according to the direction of the manufacturer.
2. Then pour olive oil in the saucepan and heat it up.
3. Add mushrooms and Italian seasonings. Stir the mushrooms well and cook for 10 minutes.
4. Then add soy milk and vegetable broth.
5. Add cooked pasta and mix up the mixture well. Cook it for 5 minutes on low heat.

per serving: 287 calories, 12.4g protein, 50.4g carbohydrates, 4.2g fat, 9g fiber, 0mg cholesterol, 26mg sodium, 74mg potassium.

Bean Hummus

Yield: 6 servings | **Prep time:** 10 minutes | **Cook time:** 40 minutes
- 1 cup chickpeas, soaked
- 6 cups of water
- 1 tablespoon tahini paste
- 2 garlic cloves,
- ¼ cup olive oil
- ¼ cup lemon juice
- 1 teaspoon harissa

1. Pour water in the saucepan. Add chickpeas and close the lid.
2. Cook the chickpeas for 40 minutes on the low heat or until they are soft.
3. After this, transfer the cooked chickpeas in the food processor.
4. Add olive oil, lemon juice, harissa, garlic cloves, and tahini paste.
5. Blend the hummus until it is smooth.

per serving: 215 calories, 7.1g protein, 21.6g carbohydrates, 12g fat, 6.1g fiber, 0mg cholesterol, 30mg sodium, 321mg potassium.

Hasselback Eggplant

Yield: 2 servings | **Prep time:** 15 minutes | **Cook time:** 25 minutes
- 2 eggplants, trimmed
- 2 tomatoes, sliced
- 1 tablespoon low-fat yogurt
- 1 teaspoon curry powder
- 1 teaspoon olive oil

1. Make the cuts in the eggplants in the shape of the Hasselback.
2. Then rub the vegetables with curry powder and fill with sliced tomatoes.
3. Sprinkle the eggplants with olive oil and yogurt and wrap in the foil (each Hasselback eggplant wrap separately).
4. Bake the vegetables at 375F for 25 minutes.

per serving: 188 calories, 7g protein, 38.1g carbohydrates, 3g fat, 21.2g fiber, 0mg cholesterol, 23mg sodium, 1580mg potassium.

Vegetarian Kebabs

Yield: 4 servings | **Prep time:** 10 minutes | **Cook time:** 6 minutes
- 2 tablespoons balsamic vinegar
- 1 tablespoon olive oil
- 1 teaspoon dried parsley
- 2 tablespoons water
- 2 sweet peppers
- 2 red onions, peeled
- 2 zucchinis, trimmed

1. Cut the sweet peppers and onions into medium size squares.
2. Then slice the zucchini.
3. String all vegetables into the skewers.
4. After this, in the shallow bowl mix up olive oil, dried parsley, water, and balsamic vinegar.
5. Sprinkle the vegetable skewers with olive oil mixture and transfer in the preheated to 390F grill.
6. Cook the kebabs for 3 minutes per side or until the vegetables are light brown.

per serving: 88 calories, 2.4g protein, 13g carbohydrates, 3.9g fat, 3.1g fiber, 0mg cholesterol, 14mg sodium, 456mg potassium.

White Beans Stew

Yield: 4 servings | **Prep time:** 10 minutes | **Cook time:** 55 minutes

- 1 cup white beans, soaked
- 1 cup low-sodium vegetable broth
- 1 cup zucchini, chopped
- 1 teaspoon tomato paste
- 1 tablespoon avocado oil
- 4 cups of water
- ½ teaspoon peppercorns
- ½ teaspoon ground black pepper
- ¼ teaspoon ground nutmeg

1. Heat up avocado oil in the saucepan, add zucchinis and roast them for 5 minutes.
2. After this, add white beans, vegetable broth, tomato paste, water, peppercorns, ground black pepper, and ground nutmeg.
3. Close the lid and simmer the stew for 50 minutes on low heat.

per serving: 184 calories, 12.3g protein, 32.6g carbohydrates, 1g fat, 8.3g fiber, 0mg cholesterol, 55mg sodium, 1011mg potassium.

Vegetarian Lasagna

Yield: 6 servings | **Prep time:** 10 minutes | **Cook time:** 30 minutes

- 1 cup carrot, diced
- ½ cup bell pepper, diced
- 1 cup spinach, chopped
- 1 tablespoon olive oil
- 1 teaspoon chili powder
- 1 cup tomatoes, chopped
- 4 oz low-fat cottage cheese
- 1 eggplant, sliced
- 1 cup low-sodium vegetable broth

1. Put carrot, bell pepper, and spinach in the saucepan.
2. Add olive oil and chili powder and stir the vegetables well. Cook them for 5 minutes.
3. After this, make the layer of sliced eggplants in the casserole mold and top it with vegetable mixture.
4. Add tomatoes, vegetable stock and cottage cheese.
5. Bake the lasagna for 30 minutes at 375F.

per serving: 77 calories, 4.1g protein, 9.7g carbohydrates, 3g fat, 3.9g fiber, 2mg cholesterol, 124mg sodium, 377mg potassium.

Carrot Cakes

Yield: 4 servings | **Prep time:** 10 minutes | **Cook time:** 10 minutes

- 1 cup carrot, grated
- 1 tablespoon semolina
- 1 egg, beaten
- 1 teaspoon Italian seasonings
- 1 tablespoon sesame oil

1. In the mixing bowl, mix up grated carrot, semolina, egg, and Italian seasonings.
2. Heat up sesame oil in the skillet.
3. Make the carrot cakes with the help of 2 spoons and put in the skillet.
4. Roast the cakes for 4 minutes per side.

per serving: 70 calories, 1.9g protein, 4.8g carbohydrates, 4.9g fat, 0.8g fiber, 42mg cholesterol, 35mg sodium, 108mg potassium.

Vegan Chili

Yield: 4 servings | **Prep time:** 10 minutes | **Cook time:** 25 minutes

- ½ cup bulgur
- 1 cup tomatoes, chopped
- 1 chili pepper, chopped
- 1 cup red kidney beans, cooked
- 2 cups low-sodium vegetable broth
- 1 teaspoon tomato paste
- ½ cup celery stalk, chopped

1. Put all ingredients in the big saucepan and stir well.
2. Close the lid and simmer the chili for 25 minutes over the medium-low heat.

per serving: 234 calories, 13.1g protein, 44.9g carbohydrates, 0.9g fat, 11g fiber, 0mg cholesterol, 92mg sodium, 852mg potassium.

Aromatic Whole Grain Spaghetti

Yield: 2 servings | **Prep time:** 5 minutes | **Cook time:** 10 minutes

- 1 teaspoon dried basil
- ¼ cup of soy milk
- 6 oz whole-grain spaghetti
- 2 cups of water
- 1 teaspoon ground nutmeg

1. Bring the water to boil, add spaghetti and cook them for 8-10 minutes.
2. Meanwhile, bring the soy milk to boil.
3. Drain the cooked spaghetti and mix them up with soy milk, ground nutmeg, and dried basil.
4. Stir the meal well.

per serving: 128 calories, 5.6g protein, 25g carbohydrates, 1.4g fat, 4.3g fiber, 0mg cholesterol, 25mg sodium, 81mg potassium.

Chunky Tomatoes

Yield: 3 servings | **Prep time:** 5 minutes | **Cook time:** 15 minutes
- 2 cups plum tomatoes, roughly chopped
- ½ cup onion, diced
- ½ teaspoon garlic, diced
- 1 teaspoon Italian seasonings
- 1 teaspoon canola oil
- 1 chili pepper, chopped

1. Heat up canola oil in the saucepan.
2. Add chili pepper and onion. Cook the vegetables for 5 minutes. Stir them from time to time.
3. After this, add tomatoes, garlic, and Italian seasonings.
4. Close the lid and sauté the meal for 10 minutes.

per serving: 550 calories, 1.7g protein, 8.4g carbohydrates, 2.3g fat, 1.8g fiber, 1mg cholesterol, 17mg sodium, 279mg potassium.

Baked Falafel

Yield: 6 servings | **Prep time:** 10 minutes | **Cook time:** 25 minutes
- 2 cups chickpeas, cooked
- 1 yellow onion, diced
- 3 tablespoons olive oil
- 1 cup fresh parsley, chopped
- 1 teaspoon ground cumin
- ½ teaspoon coriander
- 2 garlic cloves, diced

1. Put all ingredients in the food processor and blend until smooth.
2. Preheat the oven to 375F.
3. Then line the baking tray with the baking paper.
4. Make the balls from the chickpeas mixture and press them gently in the shape of the falafel.
5. Put the falafel in the tray and bake in the oven for 25 minutes.

per serving: 316 calories, 13.5g protein, 43.3g carbohydrates, 11.2g fat, 12.4g fiber, 0mg cholesterol, 23mg sodium, 676mg potassium.

Paella

Yield: 6 servings | **Prep time:** 10 minutes | **Cook time:** 25 minutes
- 1 teaspoon dried saffron
- 1 cup short-grain rice
- 1 tablespoon olive oil
- 2 cups of water
- 1 teaspoon chili flakes
- 6 oz artichoke hearts, chopped
- ½ cup green peas
- 1 onion, sliced
- 1 cup bell pepper, sliced

1. Pour water in the saucepan. Add rice and cook it for 15 minutes.
2. Meanwhile, heat up olive oil in the skillet.
3. Add dried saffron, chili flakes, onion, and bell pepper.
4. Roast the vegetables for 5 minutes.
5. Add them to the cooked rice.
6. Then add artichoke hearts and green peas. Stir the paella well and cook it for 10 minutes over the low heat.

per serving: 170 calories, 4.2g protein, 32.7g carbohydrates, 2.7g fat, 3.2g fiber, 0mg cholesterol, 33mg sodium, 237mg potassium.

Mushroom Cakes

Yield: 4 servings | **Prep time:** 15 minutes | **Cook time:** 10 minutes
- 2 cups mushrooms, chopped
- 3 garlic cloves, chopped
- 1 tablespoon dried dill
- 1 egg, beaten
- ¼ cup of rice, cooked
- 1 tablespoon sesame oil
- 1 teaspoon chili powder

1. Grind the mushrooms in the food processor.
2. Add garlic, dill, egg, rice, and chili powder.
3. Blend the mixture for 10 seconds.
4. After this, heat up sesame oil for 1 minute.
5. Make the medium size mushroom cakes and put in the hot sesame oil.
6. Cook the mushroom cakes for 5 minutes per side on the medium heat.

per serving: 103 calories, 3.7g protein, 12g carbohydrates, 4.8g fat, 0.9g fiber, 41mg cholesterol, 27mg sodium, 187mg potassium.

Glazed Eggplant Rings

Yield: 4 servings | **Prep time:** 10 minutes | **Cook time:** 10 minutes

- 3 eggplants, sliced
- 1 tablespoon liquid honey
- 1 teaspoon minced ginger
- 2 tablespoons lemon juice
- 3 tablespoons avocado oil
- ½ teaspoon ground coriander
- 3 tablespoons water

1. Rub the eggplants with ground coriander.
2. Then heat up the avocado oil in the skillet for 1 minute.
3. When the oil is hot, add the sliced eggplant and arrange it in one layer.
4. Cook the vegetables for 1 minute per side.
5. Transfer the eggplant in the bowl.
6. Then add minced ginger, liquid honey, lemon juice, and water in the skillet.
7. Bring it to boil and add cooked eggplants.
8. Coat the vegetables in the sweet liquid well and cook for 2 minutes more.

per serving: 136 calories, 4.3g protein, 29.6g carbohydrates, 2.2g fat, 15.1g fiber, 0mg cholesterol, 11mg sodium, 993mg potassium.

Sweet Potato Balls

Yield: 4 servings | **Prep time:** 15 minutes | **Cook time:** 10 minutes

- 1 cup sweet potato, mashed, cooked
- 1 tablespoon fresh cilantro, chopped
- 1 egg, beaten
- 3 tablespoons ground oatmeal
- 1 teaspoon ground paprika
- ½ teaspoon ground turmeric
- 2 tablespoons coconut oil

1. In the bowl mix up mashed sweet potato, fresh cilantro, egg, ground oatmeal, paprika, and turmeric.
2. Stir the mixture until smooth and make the small balls.
3. Heat up the coconut oil in the saucepan.
4. When the coconut oil is hot, add the sweet potato balls.
5. Cook them until golden brown.

per serving: 133 calories, 2.8g protein, 13.1g carbohydrates, 8.2g fat, 2.2g fiber, 41mg cholesterol, 44mg sodium, 283mg potassium.

Chickpea Curry

Yield: 4 servings | **Prep time:** 10 minutes | **Cook time:** 10 minutes

- 1 ½ cup chickpeas, boiled
- 1 teaspoon curry powder
- ½ teaspoon garam masala
- 1 cup spinach, chopped
- 1 teaspoon coconut oil
- ¼ cup of soy milk
- 1 tablespoon tomato paste
- ½ cup of water

1. Heat up coconut oil in the saucepan.
2. Add curry powder, garam masala, tomato paste, and soy milk.
3. Whisk the mixture until smooth and bring it to boil.
4. Add water, spinach, and chickpeas.
5. Stir the meal and close the lid.
6. Cook it for 5 minutes over the medium heat.

per serving: 298 calories, 15.4g protein, 47.8g carbohydrates, 6.1g fat, 13.6g fiber, 0mg cholesterol, 37mg sodium, 765mg potassium.

Quinoa Bowl

Yield: 4 servings | **Prep time:** 15 minutes | **Cook time:** 15 minutes

- 1 cup quinoa
- 2 cups of water
- 1 cup tomatoes, diced
- 1 cup sweet pepper, diced
- ½ cup of rice, cooked
- 1 tablespoon lemon juice
- ½ teaspoon lemon zest, grated
- 1 tablespoon olive oil

1. Mix up water and quinoa and cook it for 15 minutes. Then remove it from the heat and leave to rest for 10 minutes.
2. Transfer the cooked quinoa in the big bowl.
3. Add tomatoes, sweet pepper, rice, lemon juice, lemon zest, and olive oil.
4. Stir the mixture well and transfer in the serving bowls.

per serving: 290 calories, 8.4g protein, 49.9g carbohydrates, 6.4g fat, 4.3g fiber, 0mg cholesterol, 11mg sodium, 435mg potassium.

Vegan Meatloaf

Yield: 6 servings | **Prep time:** 10 minutes | **Cook time:** 30 minutes

- 1 cup chickpeas, cooked

- 1 onion, diced
- 1 tablespoon ground flax seeds
- ½ teaspoon chili flakes
- 1 tablespoon coconut oil
- ½ cup carrot, diced
- ½ cup celery stalk, chopped
- 1 tablespoon tomato paste

1. Heat up coconut oil in the saucepan.
2. Add carrot, onion, and celery stalk. Cook the vegetables for 8 minutes or until they are soft.
3. Then add chickpeas, chili flakes, and ground flax seeds.
4. Blend the mixture until smooth with the help of the immersion blender.
5. Then line the loaf mold with baking paper and transfer the blended mixture inside.
6. Flatten it well and spread with tomato paste.
7. Bake the meatloaf in the preheated to 365F oven for 20 minutes.

per serving: 162 calories, 7.1g protein, 23.9g carbohydrates, 4.7g fat, 7g fiber, 0mg cholesterol, 25mg sodium, 407mg potassium.

Loaded Potato Skins

Yield: 6 servings | **Prep time:** 15 minutes | **Cook time:** 45 minutes
- 6 potatoes
- 1 teaspoon ground black pepper
- 2 tablespoons olive oil
- ½ teaspoon minced garlic
- ¼ cup of soy milk

1. Preheat the oven to 400F.
2. Pierce the potatoes with the help of the knife 2-3 times and bake in the oven for 30 minutes or until the vegetables are tender.
3. After this, cut the baked potatoes into the halves and scoop out the potato meat in the bowl.
4. Sprinkle the scooped potato halves with olive oil and ground black pepper and return back in the oven. Bake them for 15 minutes or until they are light brown.
5. Meanwhile, mash the scooped potato meat and mix it up with soy milk and minced garlic.
6. Fill the cooked potato halves with mashed potato mixture.

per serving: 194 calories, 4g protein, 34.4g carbohydrates, 5.1g fat, 5.3g fiber, 0mg cholesterol, 18mg sodium, 884mg potassium.

Vegan Shepherd Pie

Yield: 4 servings | **Prep time:** 15 minutes | **Cook time:** 35 minutes
- ½ cup quinoa, cooked
- ½ cup tomato puree
- ½ cup carrot, diced
- 1 shallot, chopped
- 1 tablespoon coconut oil
- ½ cup potato, cooked, mashed
- 1 teaspoon chili powder
- ½ cup mushrooms, sliced

1. Put carrot, shallot, and mushrooms in the saucepan.
2. Add coconut oil and cook the vegetables for 10 minutes or until they are tender but not soft.
3. Then mix up cooked vegetables with chili powder and tomato puree.
4. Transfer the mixture in the casserole mold and flatten well.
5. After this, top the vegetables with mashed potatoes. Cover the shepherd pie with foil and bake in the preheated to 375F oven for 25 minutes.

per serving: 136 calories, 4.2g protein, 20.1g carbohydrates, 4.9g fat, 2.9g fiber, 0mg cholesterol, 27mg sodium, 381mg potassium.

Cauliflower Steaks

Yield: 4 servings | **Prep time:** 15 minutes | **Cook time:** 25 minutes
- 1-pound cauliflower head
- 1 teaspoon ground turmeric
- ½ teaspoon cayenne pepper
- 2 tablespoons olive oil
- ½ teaspoon garlic powder

1. Slice the cauliflower head into the steaks and rub with ground turmeric, cayenne pepper, and garlic powder.
2. Then line the baking tray with baking paper and put the cauliflower steaks inside.
3. Sprinkle them with olive oil and bake at 375F for 25 minutes or until the vegetable steaks are tender.

per serving: 92 calories, 2.4g protein, 6.8g carbohydrates, 7.2g fat, 3.1g fiber, 0mg cholesterol, 34mg sodium, 366mg potassium.

Quinoa Burger

Yield: 4 servings | **Prep time:** 15 minutes | **Cook time:** 20 minutes
- 1/3 cup chickpeas, cooked
- ½ cup quinoa, cooked
- 1 teaspoon Italian seasonings
- 1 teaspoon olive oil
- ½ onion, minced

1. Blend the chickpeas until they are smooth.
2. Then mix them up with quinoa, Italian seasonings, and minced onion. Stir the ingredients until homogenous.
3. After this, make the burgers from the mixture and place them in the lined baking tray.
4. Sprinkle the quinoa burgers with olive oil and bake them at 275F for 20 minutes.

per serving: 158 calories, 6.4g protein, 25.2g carbohydrates, 3.8g fat, 4.7g fiber, 1mg cholesterol, 6mg sodium, 286mg potassium.

Mac Stuffed Sweet Potatoes

Yield: 2 servings | **Prep time:** 20 minutes | **Cook time:** 25 minutes
- 1 sweet potato
- ¼ cup whole-grain penne pasta
- 1 teaspoon tomato paste
- 1 teaspoon olive oil
- ¼ teaspoon minced garlic
- 1 tablespoon soy milk

1. Cut the sweet potato in half and pierce it 3-4 times with the help of the fork.
2. Sprinkle the sweet potato halves with olive oil and bake in the preheated to 375F oven for 25-30 minutes or until the vegetables are tender.
3. Meanwhile, mix up penne pasta, tomato paste, minced garlic, and soy milk.
4. When the sweet potatoes are cooked, scoop out the vegetable meat and mix it up with a penne pasta mixture.
5. Fill the sweet potatoes with the pasta mixture.

per serving: 105 calories, 2.7g protein, 17.8g carbohydrates, 2.8g fat, 3g fiber, 0mg cholesterol, 28mg sodium, 308mg potassium.

Tofu Tikka Masala

Yield: 2 servings | **Prep time:** 10 minutes | **Cook time:** 25 minutes
- 8 oz tofu, chopped
- ½ cup of soy milk
- 1 teaspoon garam masala
- 1 teaspoon olive oil
- 1 teaspoon ground paprika
- ½ cup tomatoes, chopped
- ½ onion, diced

1. Heat up olive oil in the saucepan.
2. Add diced onion and cook it until light brown.
3. Then add tomatoes, ground paprika, and garam masala. Bring the mixture to boil.
4. Add soy milk and stir well. Simmer it for 5 minutes.
5. Then add chopped tofu and cook the meal for 3 minutes.
6. Leave the cooked meal for 10 minutes to rest.

per serving: 155 calories, 12.2g protein, 20.7g carbohydrates, 8.4g fat, 2.9g fiber, 0mg cholesterol, 51mg sodium, 412mg potassium.

Tofu Parmigiana

Yield: 2 servings | **Prep time:** 15 minutes | **Cook time:** 8 minutes
- 6 oz firm tofu, roughly sliced
- 1 teaspoon coconut oil
- 1 teaspoon tomato sauce
- ½ teaspoon Italian seasonings

1. In the mixing bowl, mix up, tomato sauce, and Italian seasonings.
2. Then brush the sliced tofu with the tomato mixture well and leave for 10 minutes to marinate.
3. Heat up coconut oil.
4. Then put the sliced tofu in the hot oil and roast it for 3 minutes per side or until tofu is golden brown.

per serving: 83 calories, 7g protein, 1.7g carbohydrates, 6.2g fat, 0.8 fiber, 1mg cholesterol, 24mg sodium, 135mg potassium.

Mushroom Stroganoff

Yield: 4 servings | **Prep time:** 10 minutes | **Cook time:** 20 minutes
- 2 cups mushrooms, sliced
- 1 teaspoon whole-grain wheat flour
- 1 tablespoon coconut oil
- 1 onion, chopped
- 1 teaspoon dried thyme

- 1 garlic clove, diced
- 1 teaspoon ground black pepper
- ½ cup of soy milk

1. Heat up coconut oil in the saucepan.
2. Add mushrooms and onion and cook them for 10 minutes. Stir the vegetables from time to time.
3. After this, sprinkle them with ground black pepper, thyme, and garlic.
4. Add soy milk and bring the mixture to boil.
5. Then add flour and stir it well until homogenous.
6. Cook the mushroom stroganoff until it thickens.

per serving: 70 calories, 2.6g protein, 6.9g carbohydrates, 4.1g fat, 1.5g fiber, 0mg cholesterol, 19mg sodium, 202mg potassium.

Eggplant Croquettes

Yield: 4 servings | **Prep time:** 15 minutes | **Cook time:** 5 minutes
- 1 eggplant, peeled, boiled
- 2 potatoes, mashed
- 2 tablespoons almond meal
- 1 teaspoon chili pepper
- 1 tablespoon coconut oil
- 1 tablespoon olive oil
- ¼ teaspoon ground nutmeg

1. Blend the eggplant until smooth.
2. Then mix it up with mashed potato, chili pepper, coconut oil, and ground nutmeg.
3. Make the croquettes from the eggplant mixture.
4. Heat up olive oil in the skillet.
5. Put the croquettes in the hot oil and cook them for 2 minutes per side or until they are light brown.

per serving: 180 calories, 3.6g protein, 24.3g carbohydrates, 8.8g fat, 7.1g fiber, 0mg cholesterol, 9mg sodium, 721mg potassium.

Stuffed Portobello

Yield: 4 servings | **Prep time:** 10 minutes | **Cook time:** 20 minutes
- 4 Portobello mushroom caps
- ½ zucchini, grated
- 1 tomato, diced
- 1 teaspoon olive oil
- ½ teaspoon dried parsley
- ¼ teaspoon minced garlic

1. In the mixing bowl, mix up diced tomato, grated zucchini, dried parsley, and minced garlic.
2. Then fill the mushroom caps with zucchini mixture and transfer in the lined with baking paper tray.
3. Bake the vegetables for 20 minutes or until they are soft.

per serving: 24 calories, 1.2g protein, 2.9g carbohydrates, 1.3g fat, 0.9g fiber, 0mg cholesterol, 5mg sodium, 238mg potassium.

Chile Rellenos

Yield: 2 servings | **Prep time:** 10 minutes | **Cook time:** 30 minutes
- 2 chili peppers
- 2 oz vegan Mozzarella cheese, shredded
- 2 oz tomato puree
- 1 tablespoon coconut oil
- 2 tablespoons whole-grain wheat flour
- 1 tablespoon potato starch
- ¼ cup of water
- ½ teaspoon chili flakes

1. Bake the chili peppers for 15 minutes in the preheated to 375F oven.
2. Meanwhile, pour tomato puree in the saucepan.
3. Add chili flakes and bring the mixture to boil. Remove it from the heat.
4. After this, mix up potato starch, flour, and water.
5. When the chili peppers are cooked, make the cuts in them and remove the seeds.
6. Then fill the peppers with shredded cheese and secure the cuts with toothpicks.
7. Heat up coconut oil in the skillet.
8. Dip the chili peppers in the flour mixture and roast in the coconut oil until they are golden brown.
9. Sprinkle the cooked chilies with tomato puree mixture.

per serving: 187 calories, 4.2g protein, 16g carbohydrates, 12g fat, 3.7g fiber, 0mg cholesterol, 122mg sodium, 41mg potassium.

Garbanzo Stir Fry

Yield: 4 servings | **Prep time:** 10 minutes | **Cook time:** 30 minutes
- 1 cup garbanzo beans, cooked
- 1 zucchini, diced
- 5 oz cremini mushrooms, chopped
- 1 tablespoon coconut oil

- 1 teaspoon ground black pepper
- 1 tablespoon fresh parsley, chopped
- 1 tablespoon lemon juice

1. Heat up coconut oil in the saucepan.
2. Add mushrooms and roast them for 10 minutes.
3. Then add zucchini and cooked garbanzo beans. Stir the ingredients well and cook them for 10 minutes more.
4. After this, sprinkle the vegetables with ground black pepper and lemon juice. Cook the meal for 5 minutes.
5. Add parsley and mix it up. Cook it for 5 minutes more.

per serving: 231 calories, 11.3g protein, 33.9g carbohydrates, 6.6g fat, 9.6g fiber, 0mg cholesterol, 21mg sodium, 741mg potassium.

Taco Casserole

Yield: 8 servings | **Prep time:** 10 minutes | **Cook time:** 25 minutes

- 1 teaspoon taco seasonings
- 1 cup black beans, cooked
- ¼ cup long-grain rice, cooked
- 1 zucchini, grated
- 1 cup salsa verde
- ½ cup vegan mozzarella, shredded
- 1 teaspoon olive oil

1. Brush the casserole mold with olive oil.
2. After this, mix up black beans, rice, and taco seasonings.
3. Put the mixture in the casserole molds, flatten it well, and top with salsa verde and vegan mozzarella.
4. Bake the meal at 375F for 25 minutes.

per serving: 113 calories, 6.1g protein, 19.4g carbohydrates, 1.4g fat, 4.1g fiber, 0mg cholesterol, 242mg sodium, 425mg potassium.

Chana Masala

Yield: 4 servings | **Prep time:** 10 minutes | **Cook time:** 25 minutes

- 1 cup chickpeas, cooked
- 1 jalapeno pepper, chopped
- 1 teaspoon minced garlic
- 1 teaspoon minced ginger
- 3 tablespoons fresh cilantro, chopped
- 1 tablespoon garam masala
- 1 cup tomatoes, chopped
- 1 onion, diced
- 1 tablespoon olive oil
- 2 cups of water

1. Blend together jalapeno pepper, minced garlic, ginger, and fresh cilantro.
2. Then heat up olive oil in the saucepan. Add onion and roast it until light brown.
3. Add jalapeno blend, garam masala, and chopped tomatoes.
4. Bring the mixture to boil.
5. Add chickpeas and water. Simmer the meal for 10 minutes.

per serving: 235 calories, 10.5g protein, 35.4g carbohydrates, 6.7g fat, 10g fiber, 0mg cholesterol, 23mg sodium, 606mg potassium.

Lentil Curry

Yield: 3 servings | **Prep time:** 10 minutes | **Cook time:** 25 minutes

- ½ teaspoon cumin seeds
- ¼ teaspoon coriander seeds
- 1 tablespoon coconut oil
- 1 teaspoon minced ginger
- 1 teaspoon curry powder
- 1 cup lentils
- ½ cup tomato puree
- 3 cups of water
- ½ cup of coconut milk

1. Toss coconut oil in the saucepan and melt it.
2. Add cumin seeds and coriander seeds. Bring the condiments to boil.
3. Then add minced ginger, curry powder, lentils, tomato puree, and water.
4. Bring the lentils to boil and simmer for 10 minutes.
5. Then add coconut milk and simmer the lentil curry for 10 minutes more.

per serving: 378 calories, 18.3g protein, 45.4g carbohydrates, 15.1g fat, 21.5g fiber, 0mg cholesterol, 30mg sodium, 927mg potassium.

Korma

Yield: 3 servings | **Prep time:** 10 minutes | **Cook time:** 20 minutes

- ¼ cup cashews, chopped
- 1 cup of coconut milk
- 1 cup of frozen vegetables
- 1 onion, diced
- 1 tablespoon olive oil
- 1 teaspoon garam masala

- ½ teaspoon curry powder
1. Blend together cashews and coconut milk.
2. Heat up olive oil in the saucepan and add the onion. Cook it for 3 minutes. Stir it well.
3. Then pour the mixture in the saucepan and bring it to boil.
4. Add frozen vegetables, garam masala, and curry powder.
5. Close the lid and cook korma for 10 minutes on medium heat.

per serving: 345 calories,5.8g protein, 19.7g carbohydrates, 29.2g fat, 5.7g fiber, 0mg cholesterol, 38mg sodium, 436mg potassium.

Vegan Meatballs

Yield: 8 servings | **Prep time:** 20 minutes | **Cook time:** 15 minutes
- ½ cup white beans, cooked
- ½ cup quinoa, cooked
- 2 oz vegan Parmesan, grated
- 1 oz fresh cilantro, chopped
- 1 tablespoon coconut oil
- ½ teaspoon chili flakes
- 1 tablespoon tomato paste
- ½ cup tomato puree
- 1 teaspoon ground black pepper
1. Put white beans, quinoa, and vegan parmesan in the blender.
2. Add cilantro, chili flakes, and tomato paste and blend the mixture until smooth.
3. Make the meatballs from the blended mixture and roast them in the preheated coconut oil for 3 minutes per side or until they are golden brown.
4. Then add tomato puree and ground black pepper. Close the lid and simmer the meatballs for 5 minutes on medium heat.

per serving: 109 calories,5.4g protein, 16.8g carbohydrates, 2.5g fat, 3.2g fiber, 0mg cholesterol, 27mg sodium, 397mg potassium.

Garlic Shells

Yield: 5 servings | **Prep time:** 25 minutes | **Cook time:** 15 minutes
- 10 oz jumbo shells pasta, cooked
- 1 cup marinara sauce
- 5 oz firm tofu, crumbled
- 1 teaspoon garlic powder
- ½ cup spinach, grinded
- 1 tablespoon olive oil

1. In the mixing bowl, mix up, olive oil, crumbled tofu, garlic powder, and spinach.
2. Then fill the jumbo shells pasta with garlic mixture.
3. Put the stuffed shells pasta in the casserole mold and top with marinara sauce.
4. Cover the mold with foil and bake in the preheated to 365F oven for 15 minutes.

per serving: 303 calories,10.5g protein, 49.4g carbohydrates, 6.4g fat, 3.7g fiber, 1mg cholesterol, 211mg sodium, 329mg potassium.

Seitan Patties

Yield: 3 servings | **Prep time:** 10 minutes | **Cook time:** 25 minutes
- ¼ onion, diced
- 1 bell pepper, chopped
- 8 oz seitan chunks
- 1 teaspoon coconut oil
- 1 teaspoon ground cumin
- ¼ cup oatmeal
- 1 oz walnuts, chopped
- ¼ teaspoon cayenne pepper
1. Blend together onion, bell pepper, seitan chunks, coconut oil, ground cumin, oatmeal, walnuts, and cayenne pepper.
2. When the mixture is smooth, transfer it in the bowl.
3. Preheat the oven to 365F.
4. Make 3 patties and transfer them in the lined baking tray.
5. Bake the patties for 25 minutes at 360F until they are light brown and a little bit crispy.

per serving: 522 calories,60.1g protein, 31.1g carbohydrates, 18.2g fat, 2.2g fiber, 0mg cholesterol, 3mg sodium, 178mg potassium.

Sweet&Sour Brussel Sprouts

Yield: 2 servings | **Prep time:** 10 minutes | **Cook time:** 17 minutes
- 1 cup Brussel sprouts, sliced
- 1 teaspoon liquid honey
- 1 teaspoon white pepper
- 3 tablespoons soy sauce, low-sodium
- 1 tablespoon olive oil
- 1 tablespoon pumpkin seeds, chopped
1. Heat up olive oil in the skillet.

2. Add sliced Brussel sprouts and roast them for 10 minutes. Stir the vegetables occasionally.
3. After this, sprinkle them with white pepper, soy sauce, and liquid honey. Stir the vegetables well and cook for 3 minutes.
4. Add pumpkin seeds and mix up well.
5. Cook the meal for 2 minutes more.

per serving: 109 calories, 5.3g protein, 7.7g carbohydrates, 7.3g fat, 1.9g fiber, 12mg cholesterol, 134mg sodium, 250mg potassium.

Baked Tempeh

Yield: 6 servings | **Prep time:** 10 minutes | **Cook time:** 14 minutes
- 1-pound tempeh, cubed
- ¼ cup low-sodium tamari
- 1 teaspoon nutritional yeast

1. Mix up tamari and nutritional yeast.
2. Then dip the tempeh cubes in the liquid and transfer in the lined with a baking paper baking tray.
3. Bake the tempeh for 14 minutes at 385F. Flip the tempeh cubes on another side after 7 minutes of cooking.

per serving: 154 calories, 14.8g protein, 8.3g carbohydrates, 8.2g fat, 0.2g fiber, 0mg cholesterol, 361mg sodium, 344mg potassium.

Marinated Tofu

Yield: 3 servings | **Prep time:** 20 minutes | **Cook time:** 8 minutes
- 10 oz firm tofu, cubed
- 1 tablespoon olive oil
- 1 tablespoon rice vinegar
- 1 teaspoon Italian seasonings
- 1 tablespoon marinara sauce
- 1 teaspoon coconut oil
- ½ teaspoon chili flakes

1. Make the marinade: mix up olive oil, rice vinegar, Italian seasonings, and marinara sauce. Add chili flakes and whisk the mixture gently.
2. Then sprinkle the tofu cubes with the marinade and leave for 10-15 minutes in the fridge.
3. Meanwhile, heat up coconut oil in the skillet.
4. Put the marinated tofu in the skillet in one layer and roast for 2 minutes per side or until the tofu cubes are light brown.

per serving: 132 calories, 7.8g protein, 2.5g carbohydrates, 10.7g fat, 1g fiber, 1mg cholesterol, 33mg sodium, 158mg potassium.

Zucchanoush

Yield: 6 servings | **Prep time:** 10 minutes | **Cook time:** 35 minutes
- 4 zucchinis, chopped
- 2 tablespoons olive oil
- 1 teaspoon harissa
- 1 tablespoon tahini paste
- 1 teaspoon pine nuts, roasted
- ¼ teaspoon garlic powder
- ½ teaspoon dried mint

1. Preheat the oven to 365F.
2. Put the zucchinis in the baking tray, sprinkle with olive oil and bake in the oven for 35 minutes or until the vegetables are tender.
3. Then transfer the zucchinis in the food processor.
4. Add harissa, tahini paste, pine nuts, garlic powder, and dried mint.
5. Blend the meal until smooth.

per serving: 123 calories, 3.2g protein, 8.1g carbohydrates, 10.1g fat, 2.6g fiber, 0mg cholesterol, 39mg sodium, 536mg potassium.

Garden Stuffed Squash

Yield: 2 servings | **Prep time:** 15 minutes | **Cook time:** 45 minutes
- 12 oz butternut squash, halved
- 1 bell pepper, chopped
- 5 oz leek, chopped
- 1 teaspoon dried sage
- 1 tablespoon coconut oil
- 2 oz vegan mozzarella, shredded

1. Melt the coconut oil in the skillet.
2. Add bell pepper and leek. Roast the vegetables for 3 minutes.
3. After this, add dried sage and stir well.
4. Fill the butternut squash with the vegetables mixture and top with vegan Mozzarella.
5. Bake the squash halves at 360F for 40 minutes.

per serving: 289 calories, 4.4g protein, 41.6g carbohydrates, 13.4g fat, 5.6g fiber, 0mg

cholesterol, 233mg sodium, 842mg potassium.

Broccoli Balls

Yield: 4 servings | **Prep time:** 15 minutes | **Cook time:** 10 minutes
- 1 cup broccoli, shredded
- ¼ cup quinoa, cooked
- 1 teaspoon nutritional yeast
- ½ teaspoon ground coriander
- 1 tablespoon flax meal
- 1 egg, beaten
- 2 tablespoons avocado oil

1. Mix up broccoli, quinoa, nutritional yeast, ground coriander, flax meal, and egg.
2. Stir the mixture until homogenous.
3. Then make the medium size balls.
4. Heat up avocado oil for 1 minute.
5. Put the broccoli balls in the hot avocado oil and cook them for 2 minutes per side or until light brown.

per serving: 82 calories, 4.4g protein, 9.7g carbohydrates, 3.4g fat, 2.4g fiber, 41mg cholesterol, 24mg sodium, 203mg potassium.

Vegetarian Sloppy Joes

Yield: 2 servings | **Prep time:** 15 minutes | **Cook time:** 45 minutes
- ½ cup green lentils
- 1 white onion, diced
- 1 teaspoon chili pepper
- ½ teaspoon smoked paprika
- 2 tablespoons tomato paste
- 1 tablespoon sesame oil
- 1 teaspoon liquid honey
- 2 cups of water
- ½ cup of coconut milk

1. Pour sesame oil in the saucepan.
2. Add white onion, chili pepper, smoked paprika, and cook the ingredients for 4 minutes.
3. Then add green lentils, tomato paste, liquid honey, and water.
4. Add coconut milk and stir the mixture well.
5. Close the lid and cook the sloppy joes on medium heat for 40 minutes.
6. Then remove the meal from the heat and leave it for 10 minutes to rest.

per serving: 416 calories, 15.2g protein, 43.8g carbohydrates, 21.8g fat, 18.1g fiber, 0mg cholesterol, 38mg sodium, 883mg potassium.

Tofu Stroganoff

Yield: 2 servings | **Prep time:** 15 minutes | **Cook time:** 25 minutes
- 4 oz egg noodles
- 6 oz firm tofu, chopped
- 1 tablespoon whole-wheat flour
- 1 onion, sliced
- 1 tablespoon coconut oil
- 1 teaspoon ground black pepper
- ½ teaspoon smoked paprika
- ½ cup of soy milk
- ½ cup of water

1. Roast the sliced onion with coconut oil in the saucepan until light brown.
2. Then add ground black pepper, smoked paprika, water, and egg noodles.
3. Bring the mixture to boil and cook it for 8 minutes.
4. After this, mix up flour and soy milk and pour the liquid in the stroganoff mixture.
5. Add tofu and carefully mix up the mixture.
6. Close the lid and cook tofu stroganoff for 5 minutes. Leave the cooked meal for 10 minutes to rest.

per serving: 270 calories, 12.7g protein, 28.7g carbohydrates, 12.8g fat, 3.6g fiber, 16mg cholesterol, 49mg sodium, 330mg potassium.

Turmeric Cauliflower Florets

Yield: 4 servings | **Prep time:** 10 minutes | **Cook time:** 25 minutes
- 2 cups cauliflower florets
- 1 tablespoon ground turmeric
- 1 teaspoon smoked paprika
- 1 tablespoon olive oil

1. Sprinkle the cauliflower florets with ground turmeric, smoked paprika, and olive oil.
2. Then line the baking tray with baking paper and put the cauliflower florets in the tray in one layer.
3. Bake the meal for 25 minutes at 375F or until the cauliflower florets are tender.

per serving: 50 calories, 1.2g protein, 4.1g carbohydrates, 3.8g fat, 1.8g fiber, 0mg cholesterol, 16mg sodium, 207mg potassium.

Tempeh Reuben

Yield: 4 servings | **Prep time:** 25 minutes | **Cook time:** 10 minutes
- 10 oz tempeh
- ½ cup low-sodium vegetable broth
- 1 teaspoon apple cider vinegar
- 1 teaspoon garlic powder
- 1 tablespoon olive oil

1. In the bowl mix up the vegetable broth, apple cider vinegar, and garlic powder.
2. Then put tempeh in the liquid and leave it to marinate for 15-20 minutes.
3. After this, cut tempeh into servings and put in the well-preheated skillet.
4. Add olive oil and cook it for 4 minutes per side or until golden brown.

per serving: 171 calories, 13.5g protein, 7.3g carbohydrates, 11.2g fat, 0.1g fiber, 0mg cholesterol, 47mg sodium, 302mg potassium.

Marinated Tofu Skewers

Yield: 4 servings | **Prep time:** 25 minutes | **Cook time:** 20 minutes
- ¼ cup low-fat yogurt
- 1 teaspoon curry powder
- 1 onion, diced
- 1-pound firm tofu, cubed
- ½ teaspoon chili flakes
- 1 teaspoon ground paprika

1. In the mixing bowl mix up yogurt, curry powder, onion, chili flakes, and ground paprika.
2. Then mix up yogurt mixture and cubed tofu. Leave tofu for 20 minutes to marinate.
3. After this, string the tofu cubes on the skewers and place them in the baking tray.
4. Bake the tofu for 12 minutes at 375F or until it is light brown.

per serving: 105 calories, 10.6g protein, 6.2g carbohydrates, 5.1g fat, 2g fiber, 1mg cholesterol, 26mg sodium, 265mg potassium.

Spinach Casserole

Yield: 3 servings | **Prep time:** 5 minutes | **Cook time:** 30 minutes
- 2 cups spinach, chopped
- 4 oz artichoke hearts, chopped
- ¼ cup low-fat yogurt
- 1 teaspoon Italian seasonings
- 2 oz vegan mozzarella, shredded

1. Mix up all ingredients in the casserole mold and cover it with foil.
2. Then transfer it in the preheated to 365F oven and bake it for 30 minutes.

per serving: 102 calories, 3.7g protein, 11g carbohydrates, 4.9g fat, 2.5g fiber, 2mg cholesterol, 206mg sodium, 300mg potassium.

Tofu Turkey

Yield: 6 servings | **Prep time:** 15 minutes | **Cook time:** 75 minutes
- 1 onion, diced
- 1 cup mushrooms, chopped
- 1 bell pepper, chopped
- 12 oz firm tofu, crumbled
- 1 teaspoon dried rosemary
- 1 tablespoon avocado oil
- ½ cup marinara sauce
- 1 teaspoon miso paste

1. Saute onion, mushrooms, bell pepper, rosemary, miso paste, and avocado oil in the saucepan until the ingredients are cooked (appx. 10-15 minutes).
2. Then put ½ part of tofu in the round baking pan. Press well and make the medium whole in the center.
3. Put the mushroom mixture in the tofu whole and top it with marinara sauce.
4. Add remaining tofu and press it well. Cover the meal with foil.
5. Bake the tofu turkey for 60 minutes at 395F.

per serving: 80 calories, 5.9g protein, 7.9g carbohydrates, 3.4 fat, 2.1g fiber, 0mg cholesterol, 130mg sodium, 262mg potassium.

Cauliflower Tots

Yield: 4 servings | **Prep time:** 15 minutes | **Cook time:** 20 minutes
- 1 cup cauliflower, shredded
- 3 oz vegan Parmesan, grated
- 1/3 cup flax seeds meal
- 1 egg, beaten
- 1 teaspoon Italian seasonings
- 1 teaspoon olive oil

1. In the bowl mix up shredded cauliflower, vegan Parmesan, flax seeds meal, egg, and Italian seasonings.

2. Knead the cauliflower mixture. Add water if needed.
3. After this, make the cauliflower tots from the mixture.
4. Line the baking tray with baking paper and place the cauliflower tots inside.
5. Sprinkle them with the olive oil and transfer in the preheated to 375F oven.
6. Bake the meal for 15-20 minutes or until golden brown.
per serving: 109 calories, 6.1g protein, 6.3g carbohydrates, 6.6g fat, 3.7g fiber, 42mg cholesterol, 72mg sodium, 158mg potassium.

Zucchini Soufflé

Yield: 6 servings | **Prep time:** 10 minutes | **Cook time:** 60 minutes
- 2 cups zucchini, grated
- ½ teaspoon baking powder
- ½ cup oatmeal, grinded
- 1 onion, diced
- 3 tablespoons water
- 1 teaspoon cayenne pepper
- 1 teaspoon dried thyme

1. Mix up all ingredients together in the casserole mold.
2. Flatten well the zucchini mixture and cover with foil.
3. Bake the soufflé at 365F for 60 minutes.
per serving: 41 calories, 1.6g protein, 8.1g carbohydrates, 0.6g fat, 1.6g fiber, 0mg cholesterol, 6mg sodium, 200mg potassium.

Honey Sweet Potato Bake

Yield: 4 servings | **Prep time:** 20 minutes | **Cook time:** 20 minutes
- 4 sweet potatoes, baked
- 1 tablespoon honey
- 1 teaspoon ground cinnamon
- ¼ teaspoon ground cardamom
- 1/3 cup soy milk

1. Peel the sweet potatoes and mash them.
2. Then mix mashed potato with ground cinnamon, cardamom, and soy milk. Stir it well.
3. Transfer the mixture in the baking pan and flatten well.
4. Sprinkle the mixture with honey and cover with foil.
5. Bake the meal at 375F for 20 minutes.
per serving: 30 calories, 0.7g protein, 6.5g carbohydrates, 0.4g fat, 0.5g fiber, 0mg cholesterol, 11mg sodium, 39mg potassium.

Lentil Quiche

Yield: 4 servings | **Prep time:** 15 minutes | **Cook time:** 35 minutes
- 1 cup green lentils, boiled
- ½ cup carrot, grated
- 1 onion, diced
- 1 tablespoon olive oil
- ¼ cup flax seeds meal
- 1 teaspoon ground black pepper
- ¼ cup of soy milk

1. Cook the onion with olive oil in the skillet until light brown.
2. Then mix up cooked onion, lentils, and carrot.
3. Add flax seeds meal, ground black pepper, and soy milk. Stir the mixture until homogenous.
4. After this, transfer it in the baking pan and flatten ell.
5. Bake the quiche for 35 minutes at 375F.
per serving: 351 calories, 17.1g protein, 41.6g carbohydrates, 13.1g fat, 23.3g fiber, 0mg cholesterol, 29mg sodium, 567mg potassium.

Corn Patties

Yield: 4 servings | **Prep time:** 15 minutes | **Cook time:** 10 minutes
- ½ cup chickpeas, cooked
- 1 cup corn kernels, cooked
- 1 tablespoon fresh parsley, chopped
- 1 teaspoon chili powder
- ½ teaspoon ground coriander
- 1 tablespoon tomato paste
- 1 tablespoon almond meal
- 1 tablespoon olive oil

1. Mash the cooked chickpeas and combine them with corn kernels, parsley, chili powder, ground coriander, tomato paste, and almond meal.
2. Stir the mixture until homogenous.
3. Make the small patties.
4. After this, heat up olive oil in the skillet.

5. Put the prepared patties in the hot oil and cook them for 3 minutes per side or until they are golden brown.
6. Dry the cooked patties with the help of the paper towel if needed.
per serving: 168 calories, 6.7g protein, 23.9g carbohydrates, 6.3g fat, 6g fiber, 0mg cholesterol, 23mg sodium, 392mg potassium.

Tofu Stir Fry

Yield: 3 servings | **Prep time:** 15 minutes | **Cook time:** 10 minutes
- 9 oz firm tofu, cubed
- 3 tablespoons low-sodium soy sauce
- 1 teaspoon sesame seeds
- 1 tablespoon sesame oil
- 1 cup spinach, chopped
- ¼ cup of water

1. In the mixing bowl mix up soy sauce, and sesame oil.
2. Dip the tofu cubes in the soy sauce mixture and leave for 10 minutes to marinate.
3. Heat up a skillet and put the tofu cubes inside. Roast them for 1.5 minutes from each side.
4. Then add water, remaining soy sauce mixture, and chopped spinach.
5. Close the lid and cook the meal for 5 minutes more.
per serving: 118 calories, 8.5g protein, 3.1g carbohydrates, 8.6g fat, 1.1g fiber, 0mg cholesterol, 406mg sodium, 193mg potassium.

Briam

Yield: 4 servings | **Prep time:** 20 minutes | **Cook time:** 55 minutes
- 2 zucchinis, sliced
- 2 potatoes, sliced
- 1 red onion, sliced
- 1 teaspoon dried oregano
- ½ teaspoon dried rosemary
- ½ cup fresh cilantro, chopped
- 1 cup marinara sauce
- 1 tablespoon olive oil

1. Mix up zucchinis, potatoes, and onion in the bowl.
2. Sprinkle the vegetables with dried oregano, rosemary, and cilantro.
3. Add olive oil and shake the vegetables well.
4. Then place them one-by-one in the baking pan and top with marinara sauce.
5. Cover the vegetables with foil and bake in the preheated to 385F oven for 55 minutes.
per serving: 187 calories, 4.5g protein, 31.6g carbohydrates, 5.6g fat, 6.1g fiber, 1mg cholesterol, 275mg sodium, 946mg potassium.

Dill Zucchini Patties

Yield: 6 servings | **Prep time:** 10 minutes | **Cook time:** 10 minutes
- 3 cups zucchinis, grated
- ½ cup fresh dill, chopped
- ½ cup oatmeal, grinded
- 1 tablespoon dairy-free yogurt
- 1 teaspoon ground black pepper
- 1 tablespoon canola oil

1. Mix up grated zucchini, dill, yogurt, and ground black pepper.
2. Then add oatmeal and stir the mixture until homogenous.
3. Heat up canola oil in the skillet for 2 minutes.
4. Make the patties with the help of the spoon and put them in the hot oil.
5. Cook the patties for 4 minutes per side or until patties are golden brown.
per serving: 67 calories, 2.4g protein, 9g carbohydrates, 3.1g fat, 1.9g fiber, 0mg cholesterol, 15mg sodium, 309mg potassium.

Zucchini Grinders

Yield: 2 serving | **Prep time:** 10 minutes | **Cook time:** 20 minutes
- 1 zucchini, diced
- ¼ cup marinara sauce
- 2 oz vegan mozzarella, grated
- 1 teaspoon olive oil
- 1 teaspoon chili powder

1. Roast the zucchini in olive oil for 4 minutes. Stir the vegetables occasionally.
2. After this, transfer the vegetables in the baking pan flatten well.
3. Add marinara sauce and mozzarella.
4. Cover it with foil and bake for 15 minutes at 365F.
per serving: 157 calories, 2.9g protein, 15.3g carbohydrates, 9.6g fat, 2.3g fiber, 1mg cholesterol, 361mg sodium, 380mg potassium.

Desserts

Savory Fruit Salad

Yield: 2 servings | **Prep time:** 10 minutes | **Cook time:** 0 minutes
- ½ cup strawberries halves
- ½ cup grapes, halved
- 4 oz mango, chopped
- ¼ cup fat-free yogurt
- 1 teaspoon lime zest, grated
- 1 tablespoon liquid honey

1. In the salad bowl mix up strawberries, grapes, mango, and lime zest.
2. Then add yogurt and sprinkle the salad with liquid honey.
3. Shake it gently.

per serving: 110 calories, 2.7g protein, 26.4g carbohydrates, 0.5g fat, 2g fiber, 1mg cholesterol, 25mg sodium, 279mg potassium.

Beans Brownies

Yield: 6 servings | **Prep time:** 15 minutes | **Cook time:** 15 minutes
- 1 cup black beans, cooked
- 1 tablespoon cocoa powder
- 5 oz quick oats
- 3 tablespoons of liquid honey
- 1 teaspoon baking powder
- 1 tablespoon lemon juice
- 1 teaspoon vanilla extract
- 1 teaspoon olive oil

1. Mash the black beans until smooth and mix them up with cocoa powder, quick oats, honey, baking powder, lemon juice, and vanilla extract.
2. Add olive oil and stir the mass with the help of the spoon.
3. Then line the baking pan with baking paper.
4. Transfer the brownie mixture in the baking pan and flatten it well. Cut the brownie into the bars.
5. Bake the dessert in the preheated to 360F oven for 15 minutes.
6. Cool the cooked brownies well.

per serving: 244 calories, 10.3g protein, 45.8g carbohydrates, 2.9g fat, 7.6g fiber, 0mg cholesterol, 5mg sodium, 681mg potassium.

Avocado Mousse

Yield: 2 servings | **Prep time:** 10 minutes | **Cook time:** 0 minutes
- 1 avocado, peeled, pitted
- ½ cup low-fat milk
- 1 teaspoon vanilla extract
- 1 tablespoon cocoa powder
- 2 teaspoons liquid honey

1. Chop avocado and putt it in the food processor.
2. Add milk, vanilla extract, and cocoa powder.
3. Blend the mixture until smooth.
4. Pour the cooked mousse in the glasses and top with honey.

per serving: 264 calories, 4.5g protein, 19.2g carbohydrates, 20.5g fat, 7.5g fiber, 3mg cholesterol, 34mg sodium, 653mg potassium.

Fruit Kebabs

Yield: 3 servings | **Prep time:** 10 minutes | **Cook time:** 0 minutes
- 1 cup strawberries
- 1 cup melon, cubed
- 1 cup grapes
- 2 kiwis, cubed
- 1 cup watermelon, cubed

1. String the fruits in the wooden skewers one-by-one.
2. Store the cooked fruit kebabs in the fridge, not more than 30 minutes.

per serving: 100 calories, 1.8g protein, 24.4g carbohydrates, 0.7g fat, 3.4g fiber, 0mg cholesterol, 12mg sodium, 485mg potassium.

Vanilla Soufflé

Yield: 2 servings | **Prep time:** 10 minutes | **Cook time:** 30 minutes
- 2 egg yolks, whisked
- 2 tablespoons whole-grain wheat flour
- 1 teaspoon vanilla extract
- 1 tablespoon potato starch
- 2 tablespoons agave nectar
- 1 cup low-fat milk

1. Mix up milk and egg yolks.
2. Add vanilla extract, flour, and potato starch.
3. Whisk the liquid until smooth and bring it to boil.
4. Add agave syrup and stir well.

5. Then pour the mixture into the soufflé ramekins and transfer in the preheated to 350F oven.
6. Bake soufflé for 15 minutes.
per serving: 139 calories, 7.8g protein, 12.9g carbohydrates, 5.8g fat, 0.9g fiber, 216mg cholesterol, 62mg sodium, 235mg potassium.

Strawberries in Dark Chocolate

Yield: 2 servings | **Prep time:** 15 minutes | **Cook time:** 1 minute
- 1 cup strawberries
- 1 tablespoon olive oil
- 1 oz dark chocolate, chopped

1. Melt the chocolate in the microwave oven for 10 seconds. If it is not enough, repeat 10 seconds again.
2. Then mix up chocolate and olive oil. Whisk well.
3. Freeze the strawberries for 10 minutes in the freezer.
4. Then sprinkle them with chocolate mixture.

per serving: 159 calories, 1.6g protein, 14g carbohydrates, 11.4g fat, 1.9g fiber, 3mg cholesterol, 12mg sodium, 163mg potassium.

Fruit Bowl

Yield: 4 servings | **Prep time:** 10 minutes | **Cook time:** 0 minutes
- 1 pitaya, peeled, chopped
- 2 kiwis, chopped
- 2 bananas, chopped
- ½ cup mango, chopped
- 1 teaspoon chia seeds
- 1 teaspoon coconut flakes

1. Mix up pitaya, kiwis, bananas, and mango in the big bowl.
2. Then transfer the mixture into the serving bowls and sprinkle with chia seeds and coconut flakes.

per serving: 112 calories, 1.7g protein, 26.1g carbohydrates, 1.3g fat, 3.9g fiber, 0mg cholesterol, 3mg sodium, 373mg potassium.

Berry Smoothie

Yield: 2 servings | **Prep time:** 5 minutes | **Cook time:** 0 minutes
- 1 cup blackberries
- 1 cup strawberries
- 1 cup blueberries
- 1 cup low-fat yogurt

1. Put all ingredients in the blender and blend until you get a smooth mixture.
2. Pour the cooked smoothie in the glasses.

per serving: 183 calories, 9g protein, 31.6g carbohydrates, 2.3g fat, 7g fiber, 7mg cholesterol, 88mg sodium, 569mg potassium.

Grilled Peaches

Yield: 4 servings | **Prep time:** 10 minutes | **Cook time:** 4 minutes
- 8 peaches, pitted, halved
- 1 teaspoon canola oil
- ½ teaspoon ground cinnamon

1. Preheat the grill to 395F.
2. Meanwhile, sprinkle the peaches with ground cinnamon and canola oil.
3. Put the fruits in the grill and roast them for 2 minutes per side or until the peaches are tender.

per serving: 129 calories, 2.8g protein, 28.2g carbohydrates, 2g fat, 4.8g fiber, 0mg cholesterol, 0mg sodium, 571mg potassium.

Stuffed Fruits

Yield: 3 servings | **Prep time:** 10 minutes | **Cook time:** 0 minutes
- 3 figs, raw
- 3 teaspoons low-fat goat cheese
- 1 tablespoon liquid honey
- 3 walnuts

1. Make the cross on the top of every fig and scoop a small amount of the fig meat from them.
2. Then fill the figs with low-fat goat cheese and walnuts.
3. Sprinkle the fruits with liquid honey.

per serving: 203 calories, 6.6g protein, 19.2g carbohydrates, 11.9g fat, 2.9g fiber, 15mg cholesterol, 51mg sodium, 140mg potassium.

Oatmeal Cookies

Yield: 4 servings | **Prep time:** 10 minutes | **Cook time:** 15 minutes
- 1 cup oatmeal, grinded
- 1 teaspoon vanilla extract
- 1 teaspoon honey
- 3 bananas, mashed

1. Mix up mashed bananas and oatmeal.
2. Add vanilla extract and honey. Stir the mixture well.

3. Then line the baking tray with baking paper.
4. Make the small cookies from the banana mixture with the help of the spoon and put them in the prepared baking tray.
5. Bake the cookies for 15 minutes at 360F or until the cookies are light brown.
per serving: 165 calories, 3.7g protein, 35.6g carbohydrates, 1.6g fat, 4.4g fiber, 0mg cholesterol, 2mg sodium, 393mg potassium.

Baked Apples

Yield: 3 servings | **Prep time:** 10 minutes | **Cook time:** 35 minutes
- 3 apples
- 3 pecans, chopped
- 1 tablespoon raisins, chopped
- 3 teaspoons liquid honey
- ½ teaspoon ground cardamom

1. Scoop the tops of the apples to get the medium size holes.
2. Then fill the holes with pecans, raisins, and ground cardamom.
3. Add liquid honey and wrap the apples in the foil (separately – wrap each apple).
4. Bake the apples in the preheated to 380F oven for 35 minutes.
per serving: 245 calories, 2.3g protein, 41.2g carbohydrates, 10.4g fat, 7.1g fiber, 0mg cholesterol, 3mg sodium, 327mg potassium.

Peach Crumble

Yield: 2 servings | **Prep time:** 15 minutes | **Cook time:** 25 minutes
- 1 cup peach, chopped
- 1 teaspoon ground nutmeg
- ½ teaspoon ground cinnamon
- 2 tablespoons margarine, softened
- 4 tablespoons oatmeal, grinded
- 1 teaspoon olive oil

1. Mix up margarine and oatmeal. When you get a smooth dough, crumble the mixture with the help of the fingertips.
2. After this, brush the small baking pan with olive oil and put the peaches inside.
3. Sprinkle the peaches with ground nutmeg and ground cinnamon.
4. After this, top the fruits with crumbled dough.
5. Bake the meal for 25 minutes at 360F or until you get the light brown crust.

per serving: 197 calories, 2.3g protein, 15.1g carbohydrates, 15g fat, 2.7g fiber, 0mg cholesterol, 134mg sodium, 192mg potassium.

Banana Saute

Yield: 2 servings | **Prep time:** 5 minutes | **Cook time:** 5 minutes
- 2 bananas, peeled
- 2 tablespoons orange juice
- 1 tablespoon margarine

1. Slice the bananas lengthwise.
2. Toss the margarine in the skillet and melt it.
3. Put the sliced bananas in the hot margarine and sprinkle with orange juice.
4. Saute the fruits for 2 minutes per side on medium heat.
per serving: 163 calories, 1.5g protein, 28.6g carbohydrates, 6.1g fat, 3.1g fiber, 0mg cholesterol, 68mg sodium, 456mg potassium.

Rhubarb Muffins

Yield: 4 servings | **Prep time:** 10 minutes | **Cook time:** 15 minutes
- 1 cup rhubarb, diced
- ¼ cup applesauce
- 1 egg, beaten
- 1 teaspoon baking powder
- 1 cup whole-wheat flour
- 1 tablespoon avocado oil
- 1 teaspoon lemon zest, grated
- ½ cup low-fat yogurt
- 2 tablespoons of liquid honey

1. In the mixing bowl, mix up applesauce, egg, baking powder, flour, avocado oil, lemon zest, honey, and yogurt.
2. When you get the smooth texture of the mass, add rhubarb and stir it well with the help of the spoon.
3. Preheat the oven to 365F.
4. Fill ½ part of every muffin mold with rhubarb batter and transfer them in the oven.
5. Bake the muffins for 15 minutes.
per serving: 202 calories, 6.7g protein, 38.7g carbohydrates, 2.3g fat, 1.8g fiber, 43mg cholesterol, 41mg sodium, 363mg potassium.

Poached Pears

Yield: 6 servings | **Prep time:** 5 minutes | **Cook time:** 35 minutes
- 6 pears, peeled

- 3 cups orange juice
- 1 teaspoon cardamom
- 1 cinnamon stick
- 1 anise star

1. In the saucepan mix up orange juice, cardamom, cinnamon stick, and anise star.
2. Bring the liquid to boil.
3. Add peeled pears and close the lid.
4. Cook the fruits for 25 minutes on the medium heat.

per serving: 178 calories, 1.6g protein, 45g carbohydrates, 0.6g fat, 6.8g fiber, 0mg cholesterol, 4mg sodium, 494mg potassium.

Lemon Pie

Yield: 8 servings | **Prep time:** 15 minutes | **Cook time:** 15 minutes

- 1 pie crust
- ¼ cup lemon juice
- ½ cup low-fat milk
- 3 egg yolks
- 2 tablespoons potato starch

1. Pour milk in the saucepan.
2. Add starch, egg yolks, and lemon juice.
3. Whisk the liquid until smooth.
4. Simmer it for 6 minutes. Stir it constantly.
5. Then leave the mixture for 10-15 minutes to cool.
6. Pour the lemon mixture over the pie crust and flatten it well.

per serving: 181 calories, 2.8g protein, 21.9g carbohydrates, 9.3g fat, 0.5g fiber, 79mg cholesterol, 182mg sodium, 66mg potassium.

Cardamom Pudding

Yield: 2 servings | **Prep time:** 20 minutes | **Cook time:** 10 minutes

- 1 cup of coconut milk
- 1 teaspoon agar agar
- 1 teaspoon ground cardamom
- 1 teaspoon vanilla extract
- 1 teaspoon honey

1. Pour coconut milk in the saucepan.
2. Add agar, ground cardamom, and vanilla extract. Whisk the liquid until smooth.
3. Bring it to boil and simmer for 5 minutes on the low heat.
4. Then remove the pudding from heat and leave for 10 minutes to cool.
5. Add honey and stir well.
6. Transfer the pudding in the serving cups and leave for 10 minutes in the fridge.

per serving: 296 calories, 2.9g protein, 10.7g carbohydrates, 28.7g fat, 3.1g fiber, 0mg cholesterol, 20mg sodium, 333mg potassium.

Banana Bread

Yield: 6 servings | **Prep time:** 15 minutes | **Cook time:** 45 minutes

- ½ cup low-fat sour cream
- 2 bananas, mashed
- 1 teaspoon baking powder
- 1 teaspoon apple cider vinegar
- 1 egg, beaten
- ½ cup oatmeal, grinded
- ¼ cup whole-wheat flour
- 2 tablespoons margarine, melted

1. Mix up all ingredients and whisk the mixture until smooth.
2. Then preheat the oven to 360F.
3. Pour the banana bread mixture in the loaf mold and flatten well.
4. Bake the banana bread in the oven for 45 minutes.
5. Cool the cooked bread well, remove it from the loaf mold and slice into the servings.

per serving: 166 calories, 3.4g protein, 18.9g carbohydrates, 9.2g fat, 1.9g fiber, 36mg cholesterol, 66mg sodium, 295mg potassium.

Banana Split

Yield: 2 servings | **Prep time:** 10 minutes | **Cook time:** 0 minutes

- 2 bananas, peeled
- 2 tablespoons pineapple, chopped
- 2 tablespoons low-fat yogurt
- 1 teaspoon liquid honey
- 2 tablespoons granola cereals

1. Cut every banana lengthwise and place it in the serving plates.
2. Top the fruits with granola cereals, yogurt, and pineapple.
3. Then sprinkle the bananas with liquid honey.

per serving: 149 calories, 4.5g protein, 40.4g carbohydrates, 4.3g fat, 4.6g fiber, 1mg cholesterol, 16mg sodium, 554mg potassium.

Mint Parfait

Yield: 2 servings | **Prep time:** 10 minutes | **Cook time:** 0 minutes

- *2 cups low-fat yogurt*
- *1 teaspoon liquid honey*
- *2 teaspoons lime zest, grated*
- *4 oranges, peeled and chopped*
- *1 tablespoon mint, chopped*
1. Mix up all ingredients in the bowl.
2. Then transfer the dessert in the serving bowls.

per serving: 360 calories, 17.5g protein, 63.9g carbohydrates, 3.5g fat, 9.2g fiber, 15mg cholesterol, 173mg sodium, 1257mg potassium.

Pudding Dessert

Yield: 4 servings | **Prep time:** 10 minutes | **Cook time:** 24 minutes
- *1 cup strawberries*
- *1 tablespoon honey*
- *4 eggs, beaten*
- *1 tablespoon potato starch*
- *2 cups low-fat milk*
1. In a bowl, combine the strawberries with the honey and all remaining ingredients.
2. Pour the mixture in the ramekins and transfer in the oven.
3. Bake the pudding for 24 minutes at 375F.

per serving: 152 calories, 9.9g protein, 16g carbohydrates, 5.7g fat, 0.7g fiber, 170mg cholesterol, 116mg sodium, 300mg potassium.

Vanilla Chocolate Brownie

Yield: 8 servings | **Prep time:** 10 minutes | **Cook time:** 30 minutes
- *1 tablespoon cocoa powder*
- *4 egg whites, whisked*
- *½ cup hot water*
- *1 teaspoon vanilla extract*
- *1 teaspoon baking powder*
- *1 cup whole-wheat flour*
- *2 tablespoons of liquid honey*
- *1 teaspoon margarine, softened*
- *Cooking spray*
1. In the mixing bowl, mix up all ingredients and whisk them until smooth.
2. In another bowl, combine the sugar with flour, baking powder and walnuts and stir.
3. Pour the mixture into a cake pan greased with cooking spray, flatten well, bake in the oven for 30 minutes, cool down, cut into bars, and serve.

per serving: 89 calories, 3.6g protein, 17.1g carbohydrates, 0.7g fat, 0.6g fiber, 0mg cholesterol, 24mg sodium, 128mg potassium.

Walnut Pie

Yield: 8 servings | **Prep time:** 10 minutes | **Cook time:** 25 minutes
- *3 cups almond flour*
- *1 tablespoon vanilla extract*
- *½ cup walnuts, chopped*
- *2 teaspoons baking soda*
- *1 cup low-fat milk*
- *1 egg, beaten*
- *1 teaspoon liquid honey, for decoration*
1. Mix up all ingredients except honey in the bowl and pour the mixture in the baking pan.
2. Bake the pie in the oven at 370F for 25 minutes.
3. Leave the cake to cool down, sprinkle with honey, and cut into servings.

per serving: 134 calories, 5.9g protein, 4.8g carbohydrates, 10.7g fat, 1.7g fiber, 22mg cholesterol, 340mg sodium, 96mg potassium.

Milk Fudge

Yield: 12 servings | **Prep time:** 120 minutes | **Cook time:** 7 minutes
- *1 cup low-fat milk*
- *½ cup margarine*
- *½ cup of cocoa powder*
- *1 teaspoon vanilla extract*
1. Heat up a pan with the milk over medium heat, add the margarine, stir and cook everything for 7 minutes.
2. Take this off heat, add the cocoa powder and whisk well.
3. Pour the mixture into a lined square pan, flatten ell and refrigerate in the fridge for 120 minutes.

per serving: 85 calories, 1.4g protein, 3.1g carbohydrates, 8.2g fat, 1.1g fiber, 1mg cholesterol, 98mg sodium, 125mg potassium.

Charlotte Pie

Yield: 4 servings | **Prep time:** 10 minutes | **Cook time:** 30 minutes
- *2 cups almond flour*

- *1 teaspoon baking powder*
- *½ teaspoon ground cinnamon*
- *1 tablespoon honey*
- *½ cup low-fat milk*
- *1 cup apples, chopped*
- *Cooking spray*

1. Mix up almond flour, baking powder, cinnamon, honey, and milk in the bowl.
2. Whisk the mixture well and add apples.
3. Then pour this mixture into a cake pan greased with the cooking spray, flatten well and bake in the oven at 360F for 30 minutes.
4. Cool the pie down, slice and serve.

per serving: 140 calories, 4.2g protein, 17.4g carbohydrates, 7.4g fat, 3g fiber, 2mg cholesterol, 20mg sodium, 236mg potassium.

Kiwi Salad

Yield: 8 servings | **Prep time:** 10 minutes | **Cook time:** 0 minutes

- *1 watermelon, chopped*
- *1 cup raspberries, chopped*
- *2 cups kiwis, peeled and chopped*
- *8 ounces low-fat yogurt*

1. Mix up all ingredients in the salad bowl and shake well.

per serving: 60 calories, 2.4g protein, 11.5g carbohydrates, 0.7g fat, 2.4g fiber, 2mg cholesterol, 22mg sodium, 245mg potassium.

Vanilla Cream

Yield: 4 servings | **Prep time:** 120 minutes | **Cook time:** 10 minutes

- *1 cup low-fat milk*
- *1 cup fat-free cream cheese*
- *1 teaspoon vanilla extract*
- *2 tablespoons corn starch*
- *4 teaspoons liquid honey*

1. Heat up a pan with the milk over medium heat, add the rest of the ingredients, whisk, and cook for 10 minutes on low heat.
2. Divide the mix into bowls and refrigerate the cream for 120 minutes in the fridge.

per serving: 123 calories, 10.4g protein, 16.8g carbohydrates, 1.4g fat, 0g fiber, 8mg cholesterol, 343mg sodium, 191mg potassium.

Mousse with Coconut

Yield: 12 servings | **Prep time:** 10 minutes | **Cook time:** 5 minutes

- *3 cups low-fat milk*
- *2 tablespoons coconut flakes*
- *3 tablespoons corn starch*
- *3 tablespoons of liquid honey*

1. Bring the milk to boil and add coconut flakes and corn starch.
2. Simmer the mousse for 2 minutes.
3. Cool the dessert and mix it up with liquid honey.

per serving: 53 calories, 2.1g protein, 9.8g carbohydrates, 0.9g fat, 0.1g fiber, 3mg cholesterol, 27mg sodium, 97mg potassium.

Pecan Brownies

Yield: 8 servings | **Prep time:** 10 minutes | **Cook time:** 25 minutes

- *5 pecans, chopped*
- *2 tablespoons cocoa powder*
- *2 eggs, beaten*
- *2 tablespoons margarine, softened*
- *½ teaspoon baking powder*
- *1 cup almond meal*
- *Cooking spray*

1. In your food processor, mix up all ingredients except cooking spray.
2. Then spray the square pan with cooking spray, add the brownies batter, flatten it, and transfer in the oven, bake it at 350F for 25 minutes.
3. Cool the cooked brownies and cut into bars.

per serving: 174 calories, 5g protein, 4.8g carbohydrates, 16.3g fat, 2.8g fiber, 41mg cholesterol, 49mg sodium, 205mg potassium.

Mango Rice

Yield: 4 servings | **Prep time:** 10 minutes | **Cook time:** 30 minutes

- *½ cup of rice*
- *2 cups low-fat milk*
- *1 mango, peeled and chopped*
- *1 teaspoon vanilla extract*
- *½ teaspoon ground cinnamon*

1. Bring the milk to a boil and add rice.
2. Simmer it for 25 minutes.
3. Add vanilla, cinnamon, and mango, stir and cool to the room temperature.

per serving: 190 calories, 6.5g protein, 37.5g carbohydrates, 1.7g fat, 1.8g fiber, 6mg cholesterol, 56mg sodium, 354mg potassium.

Strawberry Pie

Yield: 6 servings | **Prep time:** 10 minutes | **Cook time:** 25 minutes

- 2 cups whole wheat flour
- 1 cup strawberries, chopped
- ½ teaspoon baking powder
- ½ cup low-fat milk
- 2 tablespoons margarine, softened
- 1 tablespoon coconut flakes
- 2 eggs, beaten
- 1 teaspoon vanilla extract

1. In a bowl, combine the flour with the strawberries and all the ingredients from the list above.
2. Pour the strawberry batter in the baking pan, flatten well, and cook in the preheated to 365F oven for 25 minutes.

per serving: 228 calories, 7.1g protein, 35.2g carbohydrates, 6.2g fat, 1.7g fiber, 56mg cholesterol, 75mg sodium, 180mg potassium.

Cream Cheese Pie

Yield: 12 servings | **Prep time:** 10 minutes | **Cook time:** 25 minutes

- 2 cups whole wheat flour
- 4 tablespoons margarine, melted
- 1 cup low-fat cream cheese
- 1 teaspoon vanilla extract
- 1 egg, beaten
- 2 tablespoons of liquid honey
- 1 teaspoon baking powder

1. In a bowl, combine the flour with the margarine, and cream cheese.
2. Add egg, vanilla extract, baking powder, and honey. Stir the mixture until smooth,
3. Transfer the batter in the round pan, flatten well and bake in the oven at 350F for 20 minutes.
4. Cool the pie well.

per serving: 194 calories, 4,1g protein, 19,6g carbohydrates, 11,1g fat, 0.6g fiber, 35mg cholesterol, 108mg sodium, 97mg potassium.

Ginger Cream

Yield: 5 servings | **Prep time:** 10 minutes | **Cook time:** 0 minutes

- 3 cups non-fat milk
- 1 teaspoon ginger, ground
- 2 teaspoons vanilla extract
- 1 cup nuts, chopped

1. Blend the nuts until smooth and mix them up with ginger, milk, and vanilla extract. Stir well.

per serving: 223 calories, 9.6g protein, 14.6g carbohydrates, 14.1g fat, 2.5g fiber, 3mg cholesterol, 262mg sodium, 399mg potassium.

Raspberry Stew

Yield: 6 servings | **Prep time:** 10 minutes | **Cook time:** 10 minutes

- 16 ounces raspberries
- 2 tablespoons water
- 2 tablespoons lime juice
- ¼ teaspoon lime zest, grated
- 2 tablespoons cornstarch

1. Put all ingredients except cornstarch in the saucepan and bring to boil.
2. Add cornstarch stir until it is smooth and cook for 2 minutes more.

per serving: 51 calories, 0.9g protein, 11.8g carbohydrates, 0.5g fat, 5g fiber, 0mg cholesterol, 2mg sodium, 118mg potassium.

Melon Salad

Yield: 4 servings | **Prep time:** 4 minutes | **Cook time:** 0 minutes

- 1 cup melon, chopped
- 2 bananas, chopped
- 1 tablespoon low-fat cream cheese

1. Mix up all ingredients and transfer them to the serving plates.

per serving: 75 calories, 1.2g protein, 16.7g carbohydrates, 1.1g fat, 1.9g fiber, 3mg cholesterol, 14mg sodium, 318mg potassium.

Rhubarb with Aromatic Mint

Yield: 4 servings | **Prep time:** 10 minutes | **Cook time:** 10 minutes

- ¼ cup low-fat milk
- 2 cups rhubarb, roughly chopped
- 1 tablespoon liquid honey
- 1 tablespoon mint, chopped

1. Bring the milk to boil, add mint and rhubarb.
2. Cook the dessert for 10 minutes over the low heat.

3. Then cool the meal and add liquid honey. Stir it.
per serving: 36 calories,1.1g protein, 8g carbohydrates,0.3g fat, 1.2g fiber, 1mg cholesterol, 10mg sodium, 208mg potassium.

Lime Pears

Yield: 2 servings | **Prep time:** 10 minutes | **Cook time:** 15 minutes
- 2 teaspoons lime juice
- 1 teaspoon lime zest
- 4 pears, cored and cubed
- 1 tablespoon margarine

3. Bake the pears in the preheated to 375F oven for 15 minutes.
4. Meanwhile, melt the margarine and mix it up with line zest and lime juice.
5. When the pears are baked, sprinkle them with lime juice mixture.
per serving: 148 calories,0.8g protein, 32.5g carbohydrates,3.2g fat, 6.6g fiber, 0mg cholesterol, 37mg sodium, 251mg potassium.

Nigella Mix

Yield: 8 servings | **Prep time:** 10 minutes | **Cook time:** 10 minutes
- 4 cups mango, chopped
- 1 teaspoon nigella seeds
- 1 teaspoon vanilla extract
- ½ cup apple juice
- 1 teaspoon cinnamon powder

1. Mix up all ingredients together and transfer them in the serving bowls.
per serving: 64 calories, 0.7 protein, 14.2g carbohydrates,1g fat, 1.4g fiber, 0mg cholesterol, 2mg sodium, 155mg potassium.

Peach Stew

Yield: 4 servings | **Prep time:** 10 minutes | **Cook time:** 15 minutes
- 2 cups peaches, halved
- 2 cups of water
- 1 tablespoon honey
- 2 tablespoons lemon juice

2. Mix up all ingredients in the saucepan and simmer for 15 minutes over the low heat.
per serving: 47 calories,0.8g protein, 11.5g carbohydrates,0.3g fat, 1.2g fiber, 0mg cholesterol, 5mg sodium, 156mg potassium.

Berry Curd

Yield: 2 servings | **Prep time:** 10 minutes | **Cook time:** 10 minutes
- 2 tablespoons lime juice
- 1 tablespoon margarine
- 12 ounces blueberries
- 1 tablespoon cornstarch

1. Put all ingredients except cornstarch in the saucepan and bring to boil.
2. Then blend the berries with the help of the immersion blender and add cornstarch. Simmer the curd for 3 minutes more.
per serving: 167 calories,1.4g protein, 29.4g carbohydrates,6.3g fat, 4.2g fiber, 0mg cholesterol, 70mg sodium, 146mg potassium.

Cantaloupe Mix

Yield: 4 servings | **Prep time:** 10 minutes | **Cook time:** 0 minutes
- 2 cups cantaloupe, chopped
- 2 teaspoons vanilla extract
- 2 teaspoons orange juice

1. Mix up all ingredients in the bowl and leave for 5 minutes.
2. Then transfer the dessert in the serving plates.
per serving: 34 calories,0.7g protein, 6.9g carbohydrates,0.2g fat, 0.7g fiber, 0mg cholesterol, 13mg sodium, 217mg potassium.

Lime Cream

Yield: 4 servings | **Prep time:** 10 minutes | **Cook time:** 15 minutes
- 3 cups low-fat milk
- ½ cup lime juice
- 1 teaspoon lime zest, grated
- ½ cup agave syrup
- 2 tablespoons potato starch

1. Heat up milk and add lime zest, agave syrup, and potato starch.
2. Simmer the liquid for 5 minutes more. Stir ti constantly.
3. Then cool the milk mixture, add lime juice, and stir well.
per serving: 230 calories,6.3g protein, 49.4g carbohydrates,1.9g fat, 0.2g fiber, 9mg cholesterol, 114mg sodium, 323 potassium.

Chia and Pineapple Bowl

Yield: 4 servings | **Prep time:** 10 minutes | **Cook time:** 0 minutes
- 3 cups pineapple, peeled and cubed
- 1 teaspoon chia seeds

- *1 teaspoon fresh mint, chopped*
- *1 tablespoon liquid honey*
1. Mix up all ingredients in the big bowl.
2. Then transfer the dessert in the serving bowls.

per serving: 89 calories, 1.1g protein, 21.6g carbohydrates, 0.9g fat, 2.6g fiber, 0mg cholesterol, 2mg sodium, 150mg potassium.

Plum Stew

Yield: 4 servings | **Prep time:** 10 minutes | **Cook time:** 10 minutes

- *2 plums, pitted and chopped*
- *1 pear, cored and chopped*
- *2 tablespoons agave syrup*
- *¼ cup coconut, shredded*
- *1 tablespoon nuts, chopped*
- *1 cup of water*

1. In a pan, combine plums, pear, and water.
2. Cook the mixture for 8 minutes, divide into bowls, top with nuts, agave, coconut shred, and serve.

per serving: 97 calories, 0.9g protein, 19g carbohydrates, 2.9g fat, 2.2g fiber, 0mg cholesterol, 23mg sodium, 129mg potassium.

Citrus Pudding

Yield: 4 servings | **Prep time:** 10 minutes | **Cook time:** 15 minutes

- *2 cups orange juice*
- *2 tablespoons cornstarch*
- *¼ cup of rice*
- *¼ cup agave syrup*

1. Mix up orange juice and rice in the saucepan and bring it to boil. Simmer the mixture for 10 minutes.
2. Add rice and agave syrup and simmer the pudding for 5 minutes more.

per serving: 176 calories, 1.6g protein, 42.4g carbohydrates, 0.3g fat, 0.4g fiber, 0mg cholesterol, 16mg sodium, 274mg potassium.

Pomegranate Porridge

Yield: 2 servings | **Prep time:** 5 minutes | **Cook time:** 8 minutes

- *¼ cup oatmeal*
- *1 cup pomegranate seeds*
- *1 cup pomegranate juice*

3. Mix up oatmeal and pomegranate juice and simmer the porridge for 5 minutes.
4. Then add pomegranate seeds and stir the porridge well.

per serving: 164 calories, 1.9g protein, 37.4g carbohydrates, 0.7g fat, 1.5g fiber, 0mg cholesterol, 6mg sodium, 337mg potassium.

Apricot Cream

Yield: 4 servings | **Prep time:** 10 minutes | **Cook time:** 0 minutes

- *4 tablespoons cream cheese*
- *1 cup apricot, chopped*
- *1 teaspoon vanilla extract*

1. Blend all ingredients together until you get the creamy texture.
2. Transfer the dessert in the bowls.

per serving: 53 calories, 1.1g protein, 3.9g carbohydrates, 3.6g fat, 0.6g fiber, 11mg cholesterol, 30mg sodium, 85mg potassium.

Cardamom Black Rice Pudding

Yield: 4 servings | **Prep time:** 10 minutes | **Cook time:** 20 minutes

- *5 cups of water*
- *½ cup agave syrup*
- *2 cups wild rice*
- *1 teaspoon ground cardamom*

1. Mix up rice, water, and ground cinnamon.
2. Cook the rice for 20 minutes.
3. Add agave syrup and stir the pudding well.

per serving: 413 calories, 1.8g protein, 93.4g carbohydrates, 0.9g fat, 5.1g fiber, 0mg cholesterol, 43mg sodium, 375mg potassium.

Fragrant Apple Halves

Yield: 4 servings | **Prep time:** 10 minutes | **Cook time:** 10 minutes

- *4 apples, halved*
- *2 tablespoons chia seeds*
- *1 teaspoon vanilla extract*
- *1 teaspoon ground cinnamon*

1. Rub the apples with vanilla extract and ground cinnamon and transfer in the preheated to 375F oven.
2. Bake the apple halves for 10 minutes.
3. Then sprinkle the apples with chia seeds.

per serving: 155 calories, 1.8g protein, 34.4g carbohydrates, 2.6g fat, 8.2g fiber, 0mg cholesterol, 3mg sodium, 271mg potassium.

Appendix : Recipes Index

5-Spices Chicken Wings 68

A

Allspice Shrimps 89
Almond Cookies 23
Almond Crepes 23
Almond Porridge 22
Apple Chicken 66
Apple Oats 13
Apricot Cream 115
Aromatic Breakfast Granola 15
Aromatic Cauliflower Florets 25
Aromatic Mushroom Bowl 20
Aromatic Salmon with Fennel Seeds 89
Aromatic Whole Grain Spaghetti 94
Artichoke Chicken Stew 63
Artichoke Eggs 18
Arugula Salad with Shallot 49
Asian Style Asparagus 25
Asian Style Cobb Salad 45
Asparagus Chicken Mix 63
Asparagus Cream Soup 35
Asparagus in Sauce 29
Asparagus Omelet 14
Avocado Chicken Slices 64
Avocado Mousse 107
Avocado Salad 50
Avocado Sweet Salad 55

B

Baked Apples 109
Baked Beef Tenders 76
Baked Cod 82
Baked Falafel 95
Baked Fruits 24
Baked Herbed Carrot 28
Baked Tempeh 102
Baked Zucchini 31
Balsamic Vinegar Chicken 61
Balsamic Vinegar Salad 55
Balsamic Vinegar Steak 80
Banana Bread 110
Banana Pancakes 15
Banana Saute 109
Banana Split 110
Basil Corn 34
Basil Halibut 83
Basil Stuffed Chicken Breast 60
Basil Sweet Potatoes 32
Bean Casserole 19
Bean Frittata 14
Bean Hummus 93
Bean Sprouts Salad 53

Beans Brownies 107
Beans in Blended Spinach 33
Beans in Tahini Paste 33
Beans Mix 22
Beef Casserole 73
Beef Chili 72
Beef Ranch Steak 74
Beef Saute 75
Beef Skillet 72
Beef Soup 35
Beef Stroganoff Strips 77
Berry Curd 114
Berry Pancakes 17
Berry Quinoa 19
Berry Salad with Shrimps 50
Berry Smoothie 108
Bistro Beef Tenderloins 79
Black Beans Soup 35
Black Currant Beef Loin 80
Blackened Chicken 58
Blueberries Mix 23
Braised Artichokes 27
Braised Baby Carrot 26
Braised Seabass 84
Breakfast Almond Smoothie 14
Breakfast Splits 15
Broccoli and Cod Mash 88
Broccoli Balls 103
Brussel Sprouts Mix 25
Buckwheat Crepes 13
Buckwheat Soup 38
Butternut Squash Salad 56

C

Cantaloupe Mix 114
Cardamom Black Rice Pudding 115
Cardamom Pudding 110
Caribbean Pork Chops 79
Carrot Cakes 94
Carrot Chicken 67
Carrot Soup 36
Cauliflower Bake 30
Cauliflower Soup 38
Cauliflower Steaks 97
Cauliflower Tots 104
Cauliflower-Potato Soup 43
Celeriac Salad 48
Celery and Leek Soup 43
Celery Beef Stew 72
Celery Crab Salad 91
Celery Cream Soup 38
Chana Masala 100

Charlotte Pie 111
Cheese Hash Browns 21
Cheese Omelet 17
Cheese Soup with Cauliflower 42
Cheese&Steak Salad 46
Cherry Rice 20
Chia and Pineapple Bowl 114
Chia Oatmeal 22
Chicken and Low-fat Goat Cheese Bowl 57
Chicken and Sweet Potato Aromatic Soup 45
Chicken and Vegetables Wraps 58
Chicken Broth and Shrimps Soup 44
Chicken Chop Suey 57
Chicken Dill Soup 64
Chicken in Bell Pepper 67
Chicken Oatmeal Soup 38
Chicken Packets 57
Chicken Piccata 58
Chicken Salad in Jars 47
Chicken Skillet 56
Chicken Tomato Mix 68
Chicken Topped with Coconut 65
Chicken with Collard Greens 64
Chicken with Red Onion 65
Chicken with Vegetables 63
Chicken with Zucchini Cubes 64
Chicken-Asparagus Soup 42
Chickpea Chicken 67
Chickpea Curry 96
Chickpea Stew 28
Chile Rellenos 99
Chili Pepper Soup 44
Chili Turkey Fillet 65
Chinese Style Beef 78
Chives and Sesame Omelet 21
Chopped Chicken 67
Chunky Tomatoes 95
Cilantro Salad 51
Citrus Chicken 62
Citrus Pudding 115
Clams Stew 84
Clove Chicken 65
Cod in Orange Juice 87
Cod in Tomatoes 86
Cod in Yogurt Sauce 87
Cod Relish 85
Cold Crab Mix 90
Collard Greens Soup 43
Coriander Seafood Soup 44
Corn Patties 105
Corn Relish 26
Corn Salad with Spinach 46

Couscous Salad 48
Cranberry Pork 77
Cream Cheese Pie 113
Creamy Turkey 63
Crunchy Lettuce Salad 48
Crusted Salmon with Horseradish 81
Cucumber and Lettuce Salad 53
Cucumber and Melon Soup 36
Cucumber and Seafood Bowl 81
Cumin Cabbage 33
Cumin Chicken Thighs 68
Curries Pork 79
Curry Chicken Wings 60
Curry Pork Chops 70
Curry Snapper 84
Curry Soup 39
Curry Tofu Scramble 13

D

Dijon Potatoes 32
Dill Omelet 20
Dill Steamed Salmon 86
Dill Zucchini Patties 106
Dinner Salad 54
Dinner Shrimp Salad 55

E

Egg Toasts 16
Egg Waffles 23
Eggplant Croquettes 99
Eggs with Greens 21
Endive-Kale Salad 54

F

Fajita Pork Strips 71
Farro Salad 47
Fattoush 48
Fennel Bulb Salad 51
Fennel Pork Chops 79
Fish and Mushrooms Salad 52
Fish Salad 49
Fish Salsa 91
Fish Soup 41
Fish Spread 89
Fish Tacos 81
Five-Spices Sole 84
Fragrant Apple Halves 115
Fragrant Tomatoes 30
Fried Zucchini 32
Fruit Bowl 108
Fruit Kebabs 107
Fruit Muffins 17
Fruit Scones 17
Fruits and Rice Pudding 14

G

Garbanzo Stir Fry 99
Garden Salad 54

Garden Stuffed Squash 102
Garlic Black Eyed Peas 26
Garlic Broccoli Florets 31
Garlic Edamame Salad 54
Garlic Pork Meatballs 71
Garlic Shells 101
Garlic Soup 40
Garlic Steak 74
Ginger Cream 113
Ginger French Toast 17
Ginger Sauce Chicken 66
Glazed Chicken 62
Glazed Eggplant Rings 95
Granola Parfait 13
Grape Yogurt 19
Greek Style Salmon 88
Green Beans Soup 34
Green Cabbage Salad 55
Green Chicken Soup 44
Green Detox Soup 36
Green Dill Salad 52
Green Onion Salmon 88
Grilled Chicken Fillets 59
Grilled Cod and Blue Cheese Salad 47
Grilled Peaches 108
Grilled Pineapple Rings 28
Grilled Tilapia 86
Grilled Tofu Salad 55
Grilled Tomatoes 26
Grilled Tomatoes Soup 37
Grinded Corn 31
Ground Turkey Fiesta 73
Grouper with Tomato Sauce 84

H

Halibut with Radish Slices 88
Ham Casserole 74
Hasselback Eggplant 93
Herbed Chicken Breast 57
Herbed Melon Salad 49
Herbed Sole 82
Herbs de Provence Pork Chops 70
Hoisin Pork 72
Honey Sweet Potato Bake 105
Horseradish Cod 85
Hot Beef Strips 73

I

Iceberg Salad 51
Italian Style Zucchini Coins 27

J

Juicy Scallops 92

K

Kale and Mushrooms Soup 44
Kiwi Salad 112

L

Lean Chicken Thighs 58
Lemon Pie 110
Lemon Swordfish 83
Lemon Zest Seabass 90
Lentil Curry 100
Lentil Quiche 105
Lentil Sauté 27
Lentil Soup 37
Light Corn Stew 32
Light Shepherd Pie 75
Light Wild Rice 27
Lime Calamari 92
Lime Cream 114
Lime Pears 114
Limes and Shrimps Skewers 81
Loaded Potato Skins 97
Low Sodium Vegetable Soup 36
Low-Fat feta Hash 22
Low-Fat Sour Cream Potato 30

M

Mac Stuffed Sweet Potatoes 98
Mango Rice 112
Marinated Beef Steak Strips 78
Marinated Tofu 102
Marinated Tofu Skewers 104
Mashed Potato with Avocado 28
Meat&Mushrooms Bowl 75
Melon Salad 113
Melted Beef Bites 74
Milk Fudge 111
Milk Soup 42
Milky Mash 30
Millet Cream 22
Mint Cauliflower Salad 56
Mint Cod 86
Mint Parfait 110
Mint Seafood Salad 52
Morning Berry Salad 20
Morning Sweet Potatoes 15
Mousse with Coconut 112
Mushroom Cakes 95
Mushroom Florentine 93
Mushroom Stroganoff 98
Mustard Arctic Char 87
Mustard Tuna Salad 85

N

Nectarine Salad with Shrimps 45
Nigella Mix 114
Nutmeg Soup 41

O

Oatmeal Cookies 108
Omelet with Peppers 18
Onion and Curry Paste Chicken 68
Onion Chicken 61

Onion Omelet 24
Onion Potatoes 31
Onion Tilapia 90
Orange Mango Salad 54
Oregano Pork Tenderloin 76
Oregano Turkey Tenders 59

P

Paprika Tilapia 82
Paprika Tuna Steaks 86
Parsley Broccoli 30
Parsley Celery Root 26
Parsley Soup 39
Parsley Trout 87
Parsnip Turkey 67
Pasta Soup 35
Peach Crumble 109
Peach Pancakes 15
Peach Stew 114
Peach Turkey 62
Pecan Brownies 112
Pepper Pork Tenderloins 71
Pine Nuts Salad 53
Pineapple Porridge 23
Plum Stew 115
Poached Pears 109
Pomegranate Porridge 115
Pork Casserole 74
Pork Roast with Orange Sauce 70
Pork Sliders Meat 75
Pork Soup 39
Pork Stuffed Peppers 76
Potato Pan 29
Poultry Soup 40
Pudding Dessert 111
Pumpkin Chicken 63
Pumpkin Cream Soup 37

Q

Quinoa Bowl 28
Quinoa Bowl 96
Quinoa Burger 98
Quinoa Cakes 18
Quinoa Chicken 66
Quinoa Hashes 18
Quinoa Soup 41

R

Raspberry Stew 113
Raspberry Yogurt 16
Red Cabbage Soup 43
Red Eggplant Soup 42
Red Kidney Beans Soup 39
Rhubarb Muffins 109
Rhubarb with Aromatic Mint 113
Rice with Turkey 65
Roasted Carrot Halves 33
Roasted Tomatoes Soup 40
Rosemary Salmon 82
Russet Potato Salad 52

S

Saffron Spiced Shrimps 89
Sage Asparagus 33
Sage Beef Loin 72
Salad Skewers 45
Salmon and Corn Salad 85
Salmon in Capers 85
Salmon Salad 49
Salmon with Basil and Garlic 87
Salmon with Grated Beets 90
Salsa Eggs 16
Sausage Casserole 20
Sautéed Celery Stalk 28
Sautéed Swiss Chard 25
Savory Fruit Salad 107
Scallions Omelet 14
Scallions Risotto 19
Scallop Salad 91
Seafood Arugula Salad 50
Seafood Salad with Grapes 51
Seasoned Baked Veal 80
Seitan Patties 101
Sesame Seeds Brussel Sprouts 29
Sesame Shredded Chicken 58
Shallot Brussel Sprouts 32
Shallot Tuna 85
Shredded Beef Salad 46
Shrimp Putanesca 83
Sliced Mushrooms Salad 50
Sloppy Joe 73
Smoked Salad 50
Soft Sage Turkey 66
Southwestern Steak 70
Spanish Style Mussels 90
Spiced Baby Carrot 29
Spiced Beef 71
Spiced Eggplant Slices 27
Spiced Mushrooms 31
Spiced Scallops 83
Spiced Turkey Fillet 61
Spicy Ginger Seabass 88
Spinach and Chicken Salad 51
Spinach Casserole 104
Spinach Halibut 86
Spinach Pork Cubes 77
Spiralized Zucchini Salad 21
Spring Chicken Mix 62
Spring Greens Salad 49
Spring Salad 53
Stalk Soup 43
Strawberries in Dark Chocolate 108

Strawberry Pie 113
Strawberry Sandwich 17
Stuffed Fruits 108
Stuffed Pork Loin with Nuts 78
Stuffed Portobello 99
Stuffed Tomatoes 78
Summer Berry Soup 34
Sweet Paprika Carrot 32
Sweet Persimmon Salad 52
Sweet Potato Balls 96
Sweet Yogurt with Figs 16
Sweet&Sour Brussel Sprouts 101

T

Tabbouleh Salad 48
Taco Casserole 100
Tandoori Beef 76
Tangerine and Edamame Salad 46
Tempeh Reuben 104
Tender Endives Salad 53
Tender Green Beans Salad 51
Tender Pork Medallions 70
Thai Steak 78
Thai Style Chicken Cubes 66
Thyme Potatoes 29
Tilapia Veracruz 83
Tofu Parmigiana 98
Tofu Stir Fry 106
Tofu Stroganoff 103
Tofu Tikka Masala 98
Tofu Turkey 104
Tomato and Beef Salad 54
Tomato Bean Soup 39
Tomato Beef 71
Tomato Brussel Sprouts 30
Tomato Chicken Stew 61
Tomato Egg Whites 24
Tomato Halibut Fillets 87
Tomato Salad 46
Tropical Salad 53
Trout Soup 41
Tuna and Pineapple Kebob 81
Tuna Salad 49
Tuna Stuffed Zucchini Boats 82
Turkey and Savoy Cabbage Mix 66
Turkey Bake 59
Turkey Burgers 60
Turkey Chili 59
Turkey Meatloaf 60

Turkey Mix 61
Turkey Mushrooms 62
Turkey Soup 34
Turkey Stir-Fry 56
Turkey with Bok Choy 64
Turkey with Olives 68
Turmeric Cauliflower Florets 103
Turmeric Endives 33
Turmeric Meatloaf 73
Turmeric Pate 91

V

Vanilla Chocolate Brownie 111
Vanilla Cream 112
Vanilla Soufflé 107
Vanilla Toasts 16
Vegan Chili 94
Vegan Meatballs 101
Vegan Meatloaf 96
Vegan Salad 55
Vegan Shepherd Pie 97
Vegetable Salad with Chickpeas 19
Vegetables with Hash Browns 19
Vegetarian Kebabs 93
Vegetarian Lasagna 94
Vegetarian Sloppy Joes 103
Vinegar Trout 91

W

Walnut Pie 111
Walnut Pudding 21
Warm Lentil Salad 47
Watercress Salad 50
White Beans Stew 93
White Cabbage Rolls 76
White Mushrooms Soup 42
Whole Grain Pancakes 13
Wild Rice Soup 36

Y

Yellow Onion Soup 40
Yellow-Green Saute 31
Yogurt Shrimps 89
Yogurt Soup 41

Z

Zucchanoush 102
Zucchini Grinders 106
Zucchini Noodles Soup 37
Zucchini Soufflé 105
Zucchini Waffles 23